D1592556

The Stanford Manual
of
Cardiopulmonary Transplantation

Edited by

Julian A. Smith, M.B., M.S., FRACS
Cardiothoracic Surgeon
Deputy Head, Heart and Lung Transplant Service
Department of Cardiothoracic Surgery
The Alfred Healthcare Group
Prahran, Victoria, Australia

Patrick M. McCarthy, M.D.
Director, Implantable LVAD Program
and Heart-Lung Transplantation
The Cleveland Clinic Foundation
Cleveland, Ohio, USA

George E. Sarris, M.D.
Staff, Department of Pediatric
and Congenital Heart Surgery
Center for Pediatric and Congenital Heart Disease
The Cleveland Clinic Foundation
Cleveland, Ohio, USA

Edward B. Stinson, M.D.
Thelma and Henry Dolger Professor
Department of Cardiothoracic Surgery
Stanford University School of Medicine
Stanford, California, USA

Bruce A. Reitz, M.D.
Norman E. Shumway Professor and Chairman
Department of Cardiothoracic Surgery
Stanford University School of Medicine
Stanford, California, USA

Futura Publishing Company, Inc.
Armonk, NY

Library of Congress Cataloging-in-Publication Data
The Stanford manual of cardiopulmonary transplantation / editors,
Julian A. Smith . . . [et al.] ; with a foreword by Norman E. Shumway;
illustrations by Bayard "Butch" Colyear.
p. cm.
Includes bibliographical references and index.
ISBN 0-87993-637-1 (hardcover : alk. paper)
1. Heart—Transplantation—Handbooks, manuals, etc.   2. Lungs—
Transplantation—Handbooks, manuals, etc.   I. Smith, Julian A.
[DNLM: 1. Heart Transplantation—handbooks.   2. Lung
Transplantation—handbooks.   WG 39 S785 1996]
RD598.35.T7S73   1996
617.4'120592—dc20
DNLM/DLC
for Library of Congress   96-4754
                                                                              CIP

Copyright 1996
Futura Publishing Company, Inc.
Published by
Futura Publishing Company, Inc.
135 Bedford Road
Armonk, NY 10504
LC#: 96-4754
ISBN#: 0-87993-637-1

Dedication

This manual is dedicated to the pioneers of heart and lung transplantation—our patients and their families.

Contributors

Colleen J. Bergin, M.D. Department of Radiology, University of California, San Diego, San Diego, California

Gerald J. Berry, M.D. Department of Pathology, Stanford University School of Medicine, Stanford, California

Margaret E. Billingham, M.D. Department of Pathology, Stanford University School of Medicine, Stanford, California

Marguerite E. Brown, R.N., B.S. Department of Cardiothoracic Surgery, Bowman Gray School of Medicine, Winston-Salem, North Carolina

Ray H. Engstrom, M.D. Department of Anesthesia, John Muir Medical Center, Walnut Creek, California

David C. Fitzgerald, M.D. Department of Anesthesia, Stanford University School of Medicine, Stanford, California

Thomas F. Flavin, M.D. Cardiothoracic Consultants, P.A., Minneapolis, Minnesota

Michael B. Fowler, M.B., MRCP, FACC Division of Cardiovascular Medicine, Stanford University School of Medicine, Stanford, California

Patricia Gamberg, R.N. Department of Cardiothoracic Surgery, Stanford University School of Medicine, Stanford, California

Sharon A. Hunt, M.D. Division of Cardiovascular Medicine, Stanford University School of Medicine, Stanford, California

Anne M. Keogh, M.B., B.S., M.D., FRACP Department of Cardiology, St. Vincent's Hospital, Darlinghurst, New South Wales, Australia

Mordechai R. Kramer, M.D. Institute of Pulmonology, Hadassah University Hospital, Jerusalem, Israel

Norman J. Lewiston, M.D.†   Department of Pediatrics, Stanford University School of Medicine, Stanford, California

Sara E. Marshall, M.B, B.S., Ph.D., MRCP   Senior Registrar in Immunology, John Radcliffe Hospital, Oxford, United Kingdom

Patrick M. McCarthy, M.D.   Department of Thoracic and Cardiovascular Surgery, The Cleveland Clinic Foundation, Cleveland, Ohio

Joan Miller, R.N.   Department of Cardiothoracic Surgery, Stanford University School of Medicine, Stanford, California

Philip E. Oyer, M.D., Ph.D.   Department of Cardiothoracic Surgery, Stanford University School of Medicine, Stanford California

Peer M. Portner, Ph.D.   Baxter Healthcare Corporation, Novacor Division, Oakland, California

Bruce A. Reitz, M.D.   Department of Cardiothoracic Surgery, Stanford University School of Medicine, Stanford, California

George E. Sarris, M.D.   Center for Pediatric and Congenital Heart Disease, The Cleveland Clinic Foundation, Cleveland, Ohio

Lawrence C. Siegel, M.D.   Department of Anesthesia, Stanford University School of Medicine, Stanford, California

Julian A. Smith, M.B., M.S., FRACS   Department of Cradiothoracic Surgery, The Alfred Healthcare Group, Prahran, Victoria, Australia

Vaughn A. Starnes, M.D.   Division of Cardiothoracic Surgery, University of Southern California School of Medicine, Los Angeles, California

Edward B. Stinson, M.D.   Department of Cardiothoracic Surgery, Stanford University School of Medicine, Stanford, California

James Theodore, M.D.   Division of Pulmonary and Critical Care Medicine, Stanford University School of Medicine, Stanford, California

Randall Vagelos, M.D.   Division of Cardiovascular Medicine, Stanford University School of Medicine, Stanford, California

†Deceased

Foreword

It was the best of times. Possibly never before and probably never again will so many talented and dedicated people combine their efforts to solve, at least in part, the difficult clinical problem of cardiopulmonary transplantation. What the reader will find here is the distillation of their labors clearly and precisely written. While there are many ways to approach almost any medical challenge, the authors outline a total program for cardiopulmonary transplantation admittedly with its roots at Stanford but also with widespread successful transplantation to many other medical centers. In other words, it works.

It is essential to note that the present state of art, with respect to cardiopulmonary transplantation, evolved from the experimental laboratory. No serious thought was given to clinical application until long-term success was achieved in the laboratory. As a matter of record, one Rhesus monkey survived more than 13 years after heart-lung transplantation with minimal, essentially homeopathic, immunosuppression, and of course experiments continue to find out why. Endomyocardial biopsy was perfected in the laboratory prior to its clinical use. At the outset there was concern that the procedure might be unduly traumatic. Its fantastic benefits drove continuing investigation until clinical safety was insured.

Today it is almost trite to mention teamwork in regard to a complex clinical enterprise. Yet, a collegial atmosphere wherein mutual respect and admiration prevail is the best crucible for any transplantation program.

Norman E. Shumway, M.D., Ph.D.

Preface

The *Stanford Manual of Cardiopulmonary Transplantation* has been prepared by many of the residents and faculty involved in the care of heart and lung transplant patients during the early 1990s. The target audience is not only physicians and nurses working in a cardiopulmonary transplant unit but also medical students, house staff, other physicians, and paramedical personnel who may occasionally deal with transplant patients.

Although the patient management outlined here may not represent the only approach to heart and lung transplant patients, it does reflect the approach used by the physicians on the staff of the Department of Cardiothoracic Surgery at the Stanford University School of Medicine. Many of the methods described were pioneered at Stanford and have since achieved universal acceptance.

The emphasis of the *Manual* is on the practical day to day management of heart and lung transplant patients from the time of their initial referral through to their eventual posttransplant rehabilitation. We have attempted to present the surgical and management strategies in a clear, precise, and easily retrievable format. Some topics are controversial and are under going change, but we have endeavored to give the reader a reasonable, balanced, and safe approach to such problems.

We are indebted to the many individuals who helped bring the *Manual* to publication. We acknowledge the numerous and significant contributions of the Stanford faculty and residents who looked after the transplant patients over the years and who fostered many of developments described in the *Manual*. The excellent data collection and retrieval provided by Joan Miller, R.N. and Patricia Gamberg, R.N. is much appreciated. We are very grateful for the Herculean secretarial assistance of Marianne Brown (Cleveland Clinic Foundation) and Lynda Hudson (Alfred Healthcare Group). The outstanding illustrations created by Bayard "Butch" Colyear of the Visual Arts Service at Stanford University greatly enhance the publication.

Julian A. Smith, M.B., M.S., FRACS
Patrick M. McCarthy, M.D.
George E. Sarris, M.D.
Edward B. Stinson, M.D.
Bruce A. Reitz, M.D.

Contents

Chapter 1

Evaluating and Selecting Patients for Cardiac Transplantation

Michael B. Fowler, M.B., MRCP, FACC,
Randall Vagelos, M.D.

In 26 years of experience with cardiac transplantation at Stanford (1968–1994), various types of heart disease have been seen in patients undergoing transplantation. Ischemic heart disease (248/659 patients) and idiopathic cardiomyopathy (272/659 patients) are by far the most common types. As we gain more experience in cardiac transplantation in infants, congenital heart disease will probably expand as an indication for transplantation. However, the lack of suitable donor hearts in this age group already severely limits the number of pediatric transplantation cases that can be performed. The types of heart disease seen in patients being evaluated for cardiac transplantation are shown in Table 1. Some of the diseases will probably not be as heavily represented in the future as they have in the past, for reasons to be discussed later in this chapter.

There are no fixed criteria to definitely establish when a patient with severe heart disease becomes a suitable candidate for cardiac transplantation. The most basic considerations for selecting patients for cardiac transplantation are straightforward. First, they should be suffering from end-stage cardiac disease with significant symptoms and an estimated survival less than that expected with cardiac transplantation. All patients should be on maximal medical therapy. Next, alternative surgical therapies should already have been rejected as unrealistic. Third, candidates should be free of any extracardiac disorder that might jeopardize their postoperative survival or limit the quality of their rehabilitation. Finally, the prospective recipient must show sufficient motivation to comply with medical recommendations and to adopt an active lifestyle after transplantation. It is also important that the candidate have family, relatives, or friends to provide positive psychosocial support.

Beyond these basic considerations, however, identifying suitable can-

From: Smith JA, McCarthy PM, Sarris GE, Stinson EB, Reitz BA (eds.): The Stanford Manual of Cardiopulmonary Transplantation. Futura Publishing Co., Inc., Armonk, NY, 1996.

Table 1

Types of Cardiac Disease in a Group of 615 Candidates for Cardiac
Transplantation at Stanford

Presenting Cardiac Disease	Number of Patients
Cardiomyopathy	303
Coronary artery disease	247
Valve disease with cardiomyopathy	27
Congenital heart disease	27
Sarcoid	3
Coronary artery emboli	2
Myocarditis	2
Amyloid	1
Cardiac tumor	1
Post traumatic aneurysm	1
Marfan's syndrome	1

didates for cardiac transplantation becomes more difficult, especially with older patients. For the referring cardiologist the decision is complicated by conflicting considerations. On one hand, the results of cardiac transplantation are extraordinarily good. At present, 80%–90% of patients are alive at 1 year and approximately 65% are alive at 5 years after transplantation. On the other hand, not only are the potential costs of the operation extremely high, but the supply of donor organs is also limited. The demand for donor organs far exceeds the supply. Based on these considerations, the cardiologist who refers potential cardiac transplant candidates might follow one of two approaches, although both have real limitations for the patients involved.

If the cardiologist takes a broad approach and recommends transplantation for any patient whose left ventricular ejection fraction is < 20%, the list of patients waiting for the "lottery" of a suitable donor organ would grow unrealistically long and give many patients false hope. Some patients with severe ventricular dysfunction have surprisingly few symptoms, and therefore may experience greater morbidity after cardiac transplantation than they did before the procedure.

The cardiologist might, however, choose a narrow approach and recommend transplantation only for those patients who are clearly dying. Most of the patients in this category are hospital in-patients on intravenous inotropic drugs and vasodilator therapy. Some would be supported by an intra-aortic balloon pump (IABP) device, and a few would have totally or partially implanted left ventricular (LVAD) or biventricular assist devices (BiVAD). The disadvantage of this approach is that these patients may not receive the full benefits of long-term survival after cardiac transplantation; they may suffer relatively high morbidity and mortality preoperatively and postoperatively as a result of incipient or established secondary organ failure and a very high incidence of sepsis.

Not surprisingly, most cardiologists adopt an approach somewhere between these two extremes. An individual approach to each patient's illness and his or her expectations of the quality of life after cardiac transplantation should form the basis of every decision.

Selecting Patients for Cardiac Transplantation

Initial Evaluation

Whenever possible, an initial evaluation should consist of a full review of the entire medical record of the prospective patient. Any previous catheterization data and angiographic material should also be reviewed. At this time it is often appropriate to request the referring cardiologist to investigate the patient further. If a patient has had previous coronary bypass grafting and has significant left ventricular dysfunction, but still suffers angina as a prominent symptom, exercise stress testing with thallium scintigraphy and a repeat coronary angiogram may be performed to determine whether a revascularization procedure is still feasible. This procedure would clearly be the therapeutic option to pursue if it could be undertaken with a relatively low mortality risk as well as a reasonably optimistic chance of relieving the patient's symptoms and improving the prognosis. In this way, one donor organ could be reserved for other patients who have no alternative therapeutic option.

Progression of Disease

Acutely ill patients are the most difficult patients to evaluate. It is difficult to predict the clinical course of patients in the first few months after they present with congestive heart failure. Their condition may stabilize even after a harrowing course following acute myocardial infarction or open heart surgery. Further, their initial presentation with idiopathic dilated cardiomyopathy is often clouded by initial "misdiagnosis" of this rare condition.

The survival of patients after initial presentation in a hospital setting usually follows a biexponential course. Some patients rapidly deteriorate and die. Probably the single most useful predictor of death is the clinical "brittleness" of the patient. Patients who suffer frequent episodes of decompensation after initial stabilization have a poor prognosis. Other patients who seem "dependent" on dopamine and dobutamine (having been evaluated by cardiac catheterization, echocardiography, and instrumented with a pulmonary artery catheter) may be successfully weaned from inotropic therapy. After vasodilator therapy (usually with angiotensin converting enzyme inhibitors) has been started and diuretic therapy has been adjusted, many of these patients improve so that their previously defined NYHA Class IV status reverts to a relatively stable condition.

Morbidity, however, is highest in the first 4 months after presentation, and the initial examination must include an exhaustive survey of all factors associated with an early high mortality rate. All patients who have been weaned from inotropic support, other potential candidates with severe heart failure, and patients already accepted for cardiac transplantation are followed in a dedicated pretransplantation heart failure clinic at Stanford on a weekly basis. Table 2 outlines a simple clinical scheme to classify active transplant candidates. Category I consists of in-patients who require hospitalization for circulatory support by means of inotropic drug infusion or mechanical devices. Patients hospitalized for noncardiac complications are not included in this category since their candidacy would *de facto* be placed "on hold". Category II includes all out-patients who are further classified at Stanford according to the stability of their clinical course and level of exercise capacity, as measured by maximum oxygen consumption (VO_2). These two categories of transplant candidacy generally correspond to Status I and II, respectively, of the United Network for Organ Sharing (see Chapter 2).

Obvious candidates for cardiac transplantation in Category II (Group A) are patients who appear compliant and who are adhering well to the low salt, limited fluid diet, but who continue to experience fluid retention and demonstrate clinical right, left, or biventricular failure (or a low output state evidenced by increased fatigue, and rising BUN and creatinine levels).

Table 2
Classification Criteria for Cardiac Transplant Candidates

Category I—In-patients	Dying patients—unweanable inotropic support, low output state, IABP or LV/RV assist devices
Category II—Out-patients	
Group A	Critically ill, unstable despite optimal adjustment of therapy and good compliance
Group B	VO_2 maximum less than 14.5 mL/kg per min
Group C	VO_2 maximum greater than 14.5 mL/kg per min, but other features indicating a poor prognosis

A second group of patients, when placed in the same clinic with the same educational and emotional support, seem reasonably stable (Group B). These patients have learned to live within the limits of their symptoms but, when closely questioned, they are still severely limited by their disease. For these patients exercise testing and measurement of gas exchange are particularly useful ways to gain further insight into their management. We usually use a ramp bicycle protocol with work being progressively increased by 10 watts/minute up to maximum (symptom-limited) exercise. Most patients in this group who have maximum VO_2 of < 14.5 mg/kg per min have been placed on the active cardiac transplant waiting list.

A third group of patients (Category II, Group C) who have a maximum VO_2 of > 14.5 mL/kg per min are not immediately listed for transplantation and are followed very closely through the clinic in conjunction with their own referring physicians. They may become transplant candidates through unexplained decompensation (not due to dietary or compliance failure) or other clinical events such as episodes of ventricular tachycardia or fibrillation, or progression to Group B status.

Specific Testing

Although the clinical condition and course of patients with severe heart disease remain the major factors in determining when they become active candidates for cardiac transplantation, specific testing will also affect this decision.

Right Heart Catheterization

Patients should undergo right heart catheterization as part of their pretransplantation evaluation. At Stanford, right heart catheterization is routinely repeated if the patient has been on the transplantation waiting list more than 6 months, or if clinical events suggest a change in pulmonary vascular resistance (PVR), such as a pulmonary embolism or significant deterioration of right heart function. Also, some patients initially rejected for cardiac transplantation may fall into the acceptable range after stabilization with maximal vasodilator therapy.

Right Heart Catheterization Protocol

1. Measure the right atrial, right ventricular, pulmonary artery (PA), systolic, diastolic and mean, and pulmonary artery occlusive (wedge)

pressures (POP). Patients without coronary artery disease should
have an endomyocardial right ventricular biopsy performed at the
same time as the catheterization procedure.

2. Measure the systemic pressure with a radial artery line or small bore
catheter in the femoral artery.

3. Measure cardiac output (CO) by the Fick method. In patients with
significant tricuspid regurgitation or with low cardiac outputs, an accurate measure of the cardiac output often cannot be obtained by
thermodilution.

4. Calculate the transpulmonary pressure gradient: mean PA − POP.

5. Calculate the PVR: mean PA − POP/CO = Wood units. If the PA systolic pressure is > 45 mmHg or the PVR is > 2 wood units, nitroprusside should be infused to document the potential reversibility of
pulmonary hypertension and/or pulmonary vascular resistance.

As the patient is lying flat, the dose of nitroprusside (starting low at 12.5–24
mcg/min) can rapidly be increased to reduce the PA systolic pressure to 45
mmHg or less and to lower the PVR. If too much nitroprusside is rapidly infused, an optimal point may be missed, as the POP may fall excessively and
the cardiac output may be submaximal despite a fall in PVR.

A second more important precaution is to avoid manufacturing an acceptable PVR by reducing arterial systolic pressure below 80 mmHg. Under
this circumstance apparent acceptable reductions in the PVR are associated
with an increased incidence of acute right heart failure immediately after
transplantation and a higher first-year overall mortality rate. Occasionally,
it is useful to demonstrate reversibility of the PVR into an acceptable range
by adding a constant infusion of an inotropic drug such as dobutamine.

Cardiac Biopsy

All patients with normal coronary arteries who are being evaluated for
cardiac transplantation should have a percutaneous right ventricular endomyocardial biopsy to screen for specific primary conditions. Rarely the
endomyocardial biopsy reveals previously unexpected conditions such as
sarcoid, amyloid, or hemochromatosis. The biopsy may also provide prog-
nostic information in the acute clinical setting, where an active myocarditis
may be present. The biopsy may also have a role in assessment of prognosis
in peripartum cardiomyopathy. Patients with "granulomatous heart muscle
disease" (possibly sarcoid) have been successfully transplanted without any
obvious recurrence in the grafted heart. In these patients there was no evidence of other organ involvement with sarcoid; many had been treated with

a course of steroid therapy but without a significant change in their clinical condition.

Surprisingly, patients with amyloid are also sometimes diagnosed for the first time by means of endomyocardial biopsy; sometimes their condition is missed until the electron microscopy sections are examined. These patients continue to have a malignant clinical course even after cardiac transplantation. Our experience, like that of most others, suggests amyloid soon recurs in the grafted heart, with systemic spread and a rapid downhill course. However, there are notable exceptions, with reported instances of long-term survival after transplantation for cardiac amyloid. It is still not clear whether a possible relationship to kappa or lambda light chain in different forms of amyloid heart disease is responsible for different long-term outcomes.

Patients with Previous Malignancies

A small number of patients who have been treated for cancer with the anthracycline derivative adriamycin or radiation may present with end-stage heart failure, although they have apparently recovered from their malignancies. Clinically, these patients may have predominantly systolic dysfunction from adriamycin cardiotoxicity, diastolic dysfunction from radiation-induced fibrosis, or coronary artery disease from radiation. Often, a patient will present with a combination of all types of the devastating complications of cancer therapy. In those patients whose primary clinical finding is diastolic dysfunction, very careful evaluation should be performed to exclude treatable pericardial constriction.

A few of these cancer patients have undergone successful transplantation at Stanford. An independent consultant (not the patient's primary oncologist) should assist in documenting the disease-free status of the patient and assessing the risk of recurrence with immunosuppressive therapy. In our experience, patients who have had Hodgkin's or non-Hodgkin's lymphoma have generally done well after cardiac transplantation if they were appropriately screened and selected. Conversely, patients who have a past history of solid organ malignancies such as adenocarcinoma suffer a distressingly high incidence of disseminated recurrence when they are immunosuppressed after transplantation.

Complications of Tobacco Use

As the acceptable age of the potential cardiac transplant recipient rises, the incidence of degenerative diseases in these patients increases. Patients are often referred who have had previous peripheral bypass surgery or who have clinically significant peripheral vascular disease with symptoms of intermittent claudication. Although each patient must be evaluated on his or her merit, many have had significant tobacco toxicity from years of smoking, and their lungs are impaired by obstructive pulmonary disease and/or emphysema. On the whole, such patients have a more protracted, complicated postoperative course and often do not enjoy the same degree of physical rehabilitation as non-smoking patients. Although the potential candidacy of such patients depends on many factors, the strong adverse impact of chronic pulmonary or peripheral vascular disease must be weighed accordingly during the evaluation process.

Drug Abuse

The use of alcohol and other recreational drugs is frequently a prominent factor when young patients present with apparently idiopathic heart muscle disease. Chronic cocaine abuse can almost certainly cause a cardiomyopathy, although the precise cause-and-effect relationship is usually impossible to establish since so many other drugs are often simultaneously abused by this patient, including alcohol and the agent used to "cut" (or dilute) the cocaine.

Although we have successfully transplanted patients with significant alcohol or drug abuse problems, an especially thorough psychosocial evaluation should be performed to gauge the likelihood of successful rehabilitation. Such patients are usually not placed on an active cardiac transplantation waiting list until they have demonstrated at least 1 year of alcohol-free and drug-free compliance as outpatients in the Stanford heart failure/pretransplantation clinic. Patients who have a long history of drug or alcohol abuse, who have been unable to keep a job, and who remain medically noncompliant are incapable of the vigor and discipline needed to survive after cardiac transplantation.

Myocarditis

Occasionally, patients who are acutely ill have a right ventricular biopsy that reveals the characteristic findings of acute myocarditis. Many of these patients appear to improve either spontaneously or after therapy with prednisone and/or azathioprine. In rare instances, cardiac transplantation will be performed during the acute setting of myocarditis because the patient's condition continues to worsen and a donor heart becomes available. Very few patients are transplanted under these circumstances, but their postoperative course may be associated with a higher incidence of rejection than is seen after transplantation for chronic heart muscle disease or coronary artery disease.

Other Systemic Diseases

Patients with long-standing, insulin-dependent diabetes mellitus usually have occult or clinically manifest complications related to their diabetes at the time of referral for cardiac transplantation. Because these complications are likely to be exacerbated during steroid therapy after cardiac transplantation, these patients are not generally considered suitable candidates for cardiac transplantation. In addition, patients with systemic disorders such as autoimmune diseases or connective tissue abnormalities are likely to fare worse after transplantation than patients without these complications. Because the number of cardiac transplant candidates far exceeds the donor supply, these patients are usually not accepted as candidates.

Care of Patients Before Cardiac Transplantation

Hospital Patients

Our management strategy for all patients is to attempt to transfer them from the high risk, inotropic support group (Category I) to a more stable out-patient group (Category II) (see Table 2). Many patients are referred during a phase of acute decompensation and are initially dependent on inotropic therapy. Most of these patients can successfully be weaned to chronic oral therapy, thereby maximizing the potential to use beta-blocking drugs and especially the phosphodiesterase inhibitors. We do not consider any degree of systemic hypotension an absolute contraindication to vasodilator therapy and will maximize angiotensin-converting enzyme (ACE) inhibitor therapy except for patients with significantly rising BUN and creatinine levels, or with severely symptomatic postural hypotension. This approach seems to benefit many patients in terms of overall clinical stability and reduction in hospital admissions, despite clinical features of mild symptomatic postural hypotension. A small rise in BUN and creatinine is part of the price we accept in order to gain long-term stability, improved prognosis, and reduced symptoms associated with ACE inhibitor therapy.

Dedicated Out-Patient Clinic

A dedicated out-patient clinic is very useful for managing patients before cardiac transplantation. This clinic provides optimal educational resources to prepare patients for cardiac transplantation, and strong moral support to help maintain them during the ever-increasing wait for donor hearts. An appropriate exercise regimen is encouraged to prevent cardiac cachexia, which can severely jeopardize their postoperative recovery. Medical management is directed toward adjusting vasodilator and diuretic therapy, anti-coagulant treatment, and ensuring that the patient adheres to a low-salt diet. The intensive out-patient therapy provided by performing very frequent (usually weekly) creatinine and electrolyte screening, as well as very frequent (usually one to two weekly) clinic visits, has a major beneficial impact on the survival of patients with advanced heart failure who are candidates for cardiac transplantation. Unfortunately, such a clinic is extremely labor intensive and, to be effective, it usually requires the assistance of dedicated clinic nurses for the clinical and biochemical patient monitoring. Routine features addressed during clinic visits are summarized in Table 3.

Currently, we do not perform routine antiarrhythmic therapy although most patients have 24-hour Holter monitoring performed as part of the evaluation process. Most patients accepted or being considered for cardiac transplantation have episodes of nonsustained ventricular tachycardia recorded on their electrocardiographic recordings. Only those patients with clinical episodes associated with arrhythmia undergo formal electro-

---

Table 3
Weekly Screening Procedure for New Referrals and Patients Waiting
for Cardiac Transplantation

Clinic visit: history/physical/*education* (diet, compliance)
Serum electrolytes
BUN/creatinine levels
Digoxin levels
Antiarrhythmic drug levels
Prothrombin time (most patients routinely receiving warfarin therapy)
Liver function tests
Chest film when clinically indicated, or montly in patients receiving amiodarone
   therapy
EKG/Holter testing when clinically indicated

---

physiological evaluation, and antiarrhythmic therapy is started. If the patient remains inducible or has documented episodes of ventricular tachycardia with symptoms, usually empiric amiodarone therapy is started, with or without further electrophysiological evaluation, or, increasingly, an implantable defibrillator is placed.

Some patients who were suitable transplant candidates when they presented with ventricular fibrillation or tachycardia have had automatic implantable defibrillators placed as definitive therapy. They are therefore more likely to finally be referred for cardiac transplantation at a very late stage in the progression of their congestive heart failure. Unfortunately, secondary organ failure or intractable arrhythmias may cause death, despite a functional implantable defibrillator, before a suitable donor heart becomes available.

Complications Before Cardiac Transplantation

Certain complications in patients accepted for cardiac transplantation may result in either permanent or temporary suspension from the active cardiac transplant waiting list. Patients should be placed "on hold" if they develop any infection while waiting for cardiac transplantation. Rarely, patients who have low grade fevers during critical inotropic or mechanical support but whose blood cultures are negative may still be considered "active" candidates. However, a high percentage of these patients will subsequently prove to be septic, and death is likely in this subgroup, especially from fungal septicemia. Less critically ill patients should have any infection fully treated before they are placed on the active cardiac transplant waiting list.

Patients with advanced heart failure who develop a pulmonary infiltrate are difficult to evaluate. Whenever possible, pulmonary edema should be treated and all other causes of pulmonary infiltrates investigated. Patients whose pulmonary infiltrates are secondary to embolism represent a particularly high risk group in the posttransplantation period because of the risk of infection. Our policy at Stanford is to wait at least 2–4 months after any clinically detected pulmonary embolism before placing (or replacing) a patient on the active waiting list. At that time, the chest X-ray may continue to show a persistent but stable infiltrate at the site of the original pulmonary infarction. These patients should also have a repeat measurement of pulmonary vascular resistance (PVR) since recurrent pulmonary emboli may lead to severe irreversible pulmonary hypertension.

Unexplained anemia often occurs in severely sick patients before cardiac transplantation. All anemia should be thoroughly evaluated; however, in some cases no obvious disease process can be found and iatrogenic factors may contribute to the anemia. Patients should be screened for gastrointestinal blood loss, and any peptic ulcer should be treated fully with demonstrated complete healing before they are placed on the active transplant waiting list. Also, lower gastrointestinal blood loss from polyps or occult malignancy should be completely investigated.

Diverticulosis is a common finding in elderly patients referred for cardiac transplantation, and on its own, it is not considered a contraindication for cardiac transplantation. However, diverticulitis or recurrent sepsis from diverticular disease is a contraindication to cardiac transplantation.

Conclusions

Selecting and managing patients before cardiac transplantation remain major clinical challenges. More research is needed to define more specifically what precardiac transplantation features are likely to affect the patient's immediate postoperative survival and what features predict a poor prognosis in an individual patient being considered for cardiac transplantation (Figure 1).

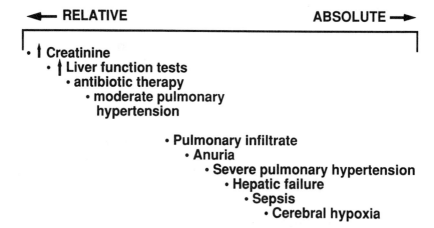

Figure 1. The decision to proceed with cardiac transplantation and the expected outcome for the patient are based on the presence of other medical conditions. The above conditions are contraindications to transplantation, and we have attempted to "rank" them according to severity. (Reproduced with permission from Vagelos/Fowler, Cardiol Clinics 1990;8:23–38.)

Appendix

Abbreviations

ACE = angiotensin-converting enzyme
BiVAD = biventricular assist device
BUN = blood urea nitrogen
CA = coronary artery
CO = cardiac output
EKG = electrocardiogram
IABP = intra-aortic balloon pump
LA = left atrial
LV = left ventricular
LVAD = left ventricular assist device
PA = pulmonary artery
PVR = pulmonary vascular resistance
POP = pulmonary artery occlusive pressure (wedge pressure)
RA = right atrial
RV = right ventricular
VO_2 max = maximum oxygen uptake during exercise testing

Selected References

1. Aravot DT, Banner NR, Khaghani A, et al. Cardiac transplantation in the seventh decade of life. Am J Cardiol 1989;63:90–93.
2. Borer JS. Determinants of prognosis in heart failure and timing of operation. Semin Thorac Cardiovasc Surg 1990;2:118–124.
3. Bourge RC, Naftel DC, Costanzo-Nordin MR, et al. Pretransplantation risk factors for death after heart transplantation: A multiinstitutional study. J Heart Lung Transplant 1993;12:549–562.
4. Costard-Jackle A, Hill I, Schroeder JS, et al. The influence of preoperative patient characteristics on early and late survival following cardiac transplantation. Circulation 1991;84 [Suppl III]:III-329-III-337.
5. Costard-Jackle A, Fowler MB. Influence of preoperative pulmonary artery pressure on mortality after heart transplantation: Testing of potential reversibility of pulmonary hypertension with nitroprusside is useful in defining a high risk group. J Am Coll Cardiol 1992;19:48–54.
6. Hildebrandt A, Reichenspurner H, Reichart B. Heart transplantation—the treatment of choice for patients with end-stage ischemic heart disease. J Thorac Cardiovasc Surg 1989;97:37–41.
7. Keogh AM, Freund J, Baron DW, et al. Timing of cardiac transplantation in idiopathic dilated cardiomyopathy. Am J Cardiol 1988;61:421.
8. Kirklin JK, Naftel DC, Kirklin JW, et al. Pulmonary vascular resistance and the risk of heart transplantation. J Heart Transplant 1988;7:331–336.

9. Lichtlen PR, Herrman G. Indications for heart transplantation in end-stage coronary disease. Adv Cardiol 1988;36:228–245.
10. Liem B, Swerdlow C. Value of electropharmacologic testing in idiopathic dilated cardiomyopathy and sustained ventricular tachyarrhythmias. Am J Cardiol 1988;62:611–616.
11. Likoff M, Chandler S, Kay H. Clinical determinants of mortality in chronic congestive heart failure secondary to idiopathic dilated or ischemic cardiomyopathy. Am J Cardiol 1987;598:634–638.
12. Massie BM, Conway M. Survival of patients with congestive heart failure: Past, present, and future prospects. Circulation 1987;75(Suppl IV):IV-11-IV-19.
13. Mudge GH, Goldstein S, Addonizio LJ, et al. Task force 3: Recipient guidelines/prioritization. J Am Coll Cardiol 1993;22:21–31.
14. Vagelos R, Fowler MB. Selection of patients for cardiac transplantation. Cardiol Clin 1990;8:23–38.

Chapter 2

Cardiac Donor Evaluation, Retrieval, and Matching to Recipient

Marguerite E. Brown, R.N., B.S.,
George E. Sarris, M.D., Philip E. Oyer, M.D., Ph.D.

As a result of clinical work in cardiac transplantation at Stanford in the 1970s, a framework of donor criteria for heart transplantation was established. Although these criteria have been extended with regard to age limits and inotropic drug support, the basic principles practiced in the 1970s of careful donor evaluation, proper size matching, and appropriate removal and preservation techniques hold true today.

Donor Evaluation

The supply of organ donors in recent years increasingly fails to keep pace with demand and has prompted transplant surgeons to carefully consider each donor referral. In the case of heart transplantation, the ability to judge donor cardiac function and predict postoperative graft performance is crucial to a successful outcome for the recipient. Donor referrals generally come from a transplant coordinator working with the local organ procurement organization. The decision to accept the heart for transplant will be made after a thorough review of clinical information. Several legal issues must also be addressed before organ recovery can take place.

Legal Criteria for Brain Death

Declaration of brain death is an absolute prerequisite to organ donation and must be carried out in accordance with state laws. Organ recovery

From: Smith JA, McCarthy PM, Sarris GE, Stinson EB, Reitz BA (eds.): The Stanford Manual of Cardiopulmonary Transplantation. Futura Publishing Co., Inc., Armonk, NY, 1996.

personnel should be familiar with the four standard clinical criteria for brain death:

Absent cortical function (unreceptivity, unresponsiveness)
Apnea
Absent brain stem function (no oculovestibular or oculocephalic re-
    flexes, no corneal, pupillary, cough, or gag reflexes)
Known cause of coma

In addition, written consent must be obtained from the appropriate next of kin. Finally, the coroner or medical examiner must be notified of the cases falling under his/her jurisdiction, and a request for organ and tissue recovery must be made.

Clinical Information

Medical History and Hospital Course

The review of donor information begins with the donor's age, sex, race, and accurate height and weight. No estimates can be taken on height and weight as this information is critical in matching donors to recipients. The transplant coordinator provides details of the mechanism of injury and the patient's clinical course from the time of injury, including pre-hospital admission events. Inquiries are made about episodes of cardiac arrest, cardiopulmonary resuscitation, hypotension, hypoxemia, arrhythmias, and thoracic trauma. If a cardiac arrest did occur, a detailed account of the event is obtained, including duration, drugs administered, and use of electroshock.

Relevant past medical history and information regarding social habits are also obtained, and any drug use, smoking, alcohol consumption, and sexual practice are noted. Cardiac disease risk factors, including family history, obesity, hypertension, diabetes, and smoking are especially relevant in assessing male donors over age 35.

To avoid any misconceptions about a donor's clinical course or history, one should consistently ask about cardiac-related issues. All cardiac information should always be confirmed through direct inquiry.

Hemodynamic Status

The use of cardioactive agents, such as dopamine hydrochloride, is noted. The amount of drug, duration of use, and relative intravascular volume status are critical in making an assessment of cardiac function. The insertion of a central venous catheter and accurate intake and output records are extremely helpful in determining the volume status. In general, if dopamine requirements exceed 10 mcg/kg per min with a normal right atrial filling pressure (central venous pressure [CVP]: 6–12 mmHg) the donor may not be suitable for heart recovery. Cardiac dysfunction may have occurred through chest trauma, resuscitative efforts, long-term pressor support, hypoxemia, or cardiac changes resulting from brain death. In some circumstances, the insertion of a Swan-Ganz catheter will provide definitive information about cardiac output and systemic resistance. Donors with high outputs and low peripheral resistance may require a small amount of neosynephrine, metaraminol (Aramine), or norepinephrine (Levophed) to restore normal vasomotor tone.

Cardiac Studies

A 12-lead electrocardiogram (EKG) and echocardiogram are routinely ordered to assess cardiac anatomy and function. It is rare to find a completely normal 12-lead interpretation on a brain-dead patient. Most donors will have nonspecific ST and T wave changes with major central nervous system damage. Other insignificant changes may be due to hypothermia and electrolyte imbalances. The presence of pathological Q waves is a contraindication to heart recovery.

Over the last several years, it has become standard practice to obtain echocardiograms on potential heart donors. It is particularly important for those donors who have had cardiopulmonary resuscitation or chest trauma. The typical assessments may include valvular appearance, chamber sizes, ventricular and septal wall motion, and estimated ejection fraction. If possible, the echocardiogram should be obtained with minimal dopamine support (< 10 mcg/kg per min). Slight abnormalities, such as mild septal hypokinesis, mitral valve prolapse with trace to mild regurgitation, or small pericardial effusions will not preclude heart recovery. Coronary arteriograms are indicated for male donors over 35 with significant cardiac risk factors. Recently, otherwise suitable donors as old as 60 years of age have been accepted. In most of these cases, a normal coronary arteriogram is a necessary prerequisite. If angiography of the donor is not possible at the donor hospital, the recipient's status and need for urgent transplantation will have some bearing on the decision to use the heart without such data.

A chest film is routinely ordered to evaluate the appearance of the heart and thorax. In some cases, the size of the heart will be measured to assure that it is the proper size to match the recipient's heart.

Laboratory Results

1. Current electrolyte results are reviewed including sodium levels and, in particular, potassium levels. Potassium replacement is given to maintain levels of 4.0–4.5 mEq/L.
2. Hematology data, such as white blood cell count, hematocrit, and hemoglobin, are noted. In general, the hematocrit is maintained above 30% with appropriate transfusions. Cytomegalovirus (CMV) negative blood (if possible), should be used if the recipient is CMV negative.
3. Arterial blood gases and corresponding ventilator settings are obtained. Adjustments are made to maintain a normal pH and adequate oxygenation.

Serology Testing Information

The final information needed from a donor before heart recovery is often the serology test results. The standard serology tests performed on organ donors include the following:

- HBsAg = hepatitis B surface antigen.
- Anti-HBs = antibody to hepatitis B surface antigen.
- Anti-HBc = antibody to hepatitis B core antigen.
- Anti-HIV = antibody to human immunodeficiency virus.
- CMV = cytomegalovirus titer.
- Hepatitis C antibody.

Positive results for the HBsAg and anti-HIV tests would rule out the use of a donor at Stanford. Positive anti-HBc results require careful considerations of donor history and risk factors for hepatitis. If possible, consideration is given to matching CMV-negative donors to CMV-negative recipients, but a mismatch will not preclude use of the heart. Although the importance of antibody to hepatitis C is not yet firmly established, a positive result for hepatitis C antibody would also exclude the use of the donor at Stanford.

Acceptable Cardiac Donor Criteria

As a general guideline, donors are suitable for heart recovery if they prove to be free of significant cardiac disease and/or injury, as best determined by history, echocardiography, ECG, and, if indicated, coronary angiography. The age of the donor may extend from newborns to age 60. The upper age limit varies from one transplantation center to another; however, careful, extensive evaluation occurs with all donors over 40 years of age.

The critical shortage of organ donors and the status of the transplant candidate will have a major impact on the decision to accept a particular donor. Also, recovery of hearts for transplantation is limited by the distance to the donor hospital and the resulting graft ischemic time. On average, ischemic times of 4–5 hours are considered the upper limit for cardiac grafts. The exception to this practice is in children and, in particular, in infant donors, where ischemic times may extend up to 8 hours with normal postoperative function.

Inotropic drug support is the area where it is most difficult to apply firm criteria. Ideally, cardiac donors should be receiving minimal dopamine dosages (3–5 mcg/kg per min). The upper limit of acceptable dopamine dependency is generally 10 mcg/kg per min, but this criterion may vary according to the donor's age, clinical course, hemodynamic data, length of time on dopamine, and the projected ischemia time for the graft.

Donors who are considered marginally suitable as a result of reports of cardiac evaluations and hemodynamic status may still prove to be acceptable after the recovery team has performed an on-site assessment.

Clinical Donor Management

Clinical management of the donor is generally accomplished through coordinators working with the local procurement organization. The goal is to provide optimal organ perfusion and oxygenation. All medical personnel involved with organ recovery must be familiar with the physiologic traits of brain-dead patients and the type of clinical interventions necessary to maintain hemodynamic stability (Table 1).

Table 1

Clinical Interventions in Donor Management*

Physiologic Consequences of Brain Death	Clinical Problem	Intervention
Loss of vasomotor tone	Hypotension	1) Restore volume (maintain CVP 5–12 cm H_2O) 2) Administer dopamine ≥ 10 mcg/kg per min (maintain systolic BP ≥ 100 mmHg) 3) Use neosynephrine, or metaraminol if needed
Hypothalamic dysfunction	Hypothermia	1) Use warming blankets, lights 2) Warm IV fluid, inspired gases (maintain temperature 36.6°–37.5°)
	Diabetes insipidus	1) Give IV fluid to match urinary output, cc/cc plus 50 cc/hr 2) Administer aqueous vasopressin (or DDAVP) 3) Monitor electrolytes every 4 hours
Pulmonary complications	Apnea	1) Use volume cycled ventilator 2) Deliver lowest F_iO_2 to maintain PO_2 ≥ 100 3) Use a tidal volume of 10–15 cc/kg, 5cm PEEP
Infection	Pulmonary	1) Perform hourly bagging and suctioning using meticulous sterile technique 2) Administer broad spectrum antibiotics
	Neurologic pulmonary edema	1) Increase inspired oxygen and PEEP as necessary to keep PO_2 > 100 2) Report condition to transplant coordinator for expeditious organ recovery 3) Monitor ABGs every 4 hours

*Guidelines for Donor Management, Department of Cardiovascular Surgery, Stanford University Medical Center, Stanford, California

Matching Donor to Recipient

Local and National Heart Allocation Systems

Offers may come to a transplantation center from local as well as distant organ procurement networks. Each transplant candidate's name, age, sex, and blood type are entered into the United Network for Organ Sharing (UNOS) computer. In addition, a suitable range is listed for the donor's height and weight, along with a recovery distance.

Patients are categorized as Status I or Status II. Status I patients must be in an intensive care unit (ICU) and have one or more of the following measures in place for their support: inotropic drug infusion to maintain adequate blood pressure and cardiac output; mechanical ventilation; intra-aortic balloon pump; and/or ventricular assist device. Status II patients include all other patients waiting at home or in hospital settings without the need for the support systems listed above.

Local registration of transplant candidates waiting for a donor varies as to the type of information each requires. The California Transplant Donor Network is the local procurement organization associated with Stanford and currently serves three heart transplant centers in the area. This network maintains one list for all patients waiting for heart transplant; this list conforms to UNOS rules about the status of waiting patients.

When a donor heart becomes available, the center listing a Status I recipient for the longest period of time is offered the heart first. Should the donor not be acceptable (usually because of size disparities), the center with the next patient on the waiting list next gets the donor option. If all Status I patients are considered unsuitable for the donor, the possibility of heart-lung recovery is explored. If the donor does not qualify, the heart is offered to the Status II patient who has waited the longest time and has the same ABO blood group (Table 2). If this recipient is not suitable for the

Table 2
Frequency of ABO Blood Types in the United States

ABO Blood Type	Western European Descent (%)	African Descent (%)
A	45	29
B	8	17
AB "Universal Recipient"	4	4
O "Universal Donor"	43	50

Modified and reproduced with permission from *Harrison's Principles of Internal Medicine.* Twelfth Edition. Wilson JD, Braunwald E, Isselbacher KJM, Petersdorf RG, Martin JB, Fauci AS, Root RK, eds. New York, McGraw-Hill, 1991, p. 1495.

donor, the center with the next patient on the waiting list then receives the offer.

Because this system is patient driven rather than center driven, it gives each patient an equal chance to receive a donor organ regardless of the length of a waiting list at any one center within the local procurement organization.

Size-Matching

The donor's height and weight are critical information needed to determine a proper size match for a recipient. A disparity in the donor's weight 20% below the recipient's weight is the lower limit for patients with a normal right pulmonary vein (PVR). For example, a patient weighing 200 lbs whose PVR of 2.0 falls to 1.5 with nitroprusside may satisfactorily accept a donor weighing approximately 160 lbs (20% of 200 lbs = 40 lbs, 200 − 40 = 160 lbs). The height, sex, and age of the donor may also be factors in determining the capacity of the donor heart.

Patients with a high PVR and high pulmonary pressures should receive donors who match or exceed the recipient's weight. Careful consideration should be given to the donor's lean body mass; which may be underestimated in the shorter, obese individual.

Cross-Matching

All patients awaiting cardiac transplantation are tested against a random panel of 50 lymphocyte donors for the presence of preformed antibodies. Most patients will exhibit no such antibodies and, therefore, generally do not require a prospective donor-specific cross-match. For those patients who show presensitization ($>$ 10% preformed antibodies), a prospective lymphocyte cross-match is usually required. Patients in this category often are women who have borne children, patients who have received multiple transfusions, and those who have received procainamide.

Organ Recovery

Donor Team Transport

At Stanford, the donor transplant team includes a resident anesthesiologist, an operating room scrub nurse, an experienced cardiac surgery resident, an assistant (who may be a medical student, intern, or surgery resident), and the donor coordinator. Other programs send fewer individuals for routine heart retrieval. The distance to the donor hospital determines whether an ambulance, helicopter, fixed-wing, or jet aircraft is needed. The donor coordinator contacts the other team members to give them approximate departure times. A call is made to the critical care transport department, and the dispatcher in this area notifies the appropriate transportation companies.

Equipment

Table 3 lists the standard equipment taken to recover the donor heart. Two metal suitcases hold these supplies and a sterile container for the heart. In addition, an igloo cooler filled with ice is packed with 3–4 liters of normal saline in pour bottles and two 500 cc bags of cardioplegia solution. A sternal saw is taken to those hospitals where cardiac surgery is not performed.

Intravenous fluids, medications (dopamine, nitroprusside, and metaraminol), central and arterial lines, dial-a-flow lines, ambu bag, and other equipment helpful to the anesthesiologist are also taken to reduce impositions on the donor hospital staff.

Table 3
Supplies Used for Cardiectomy of the Donor Heart

1	#5 wire
2	#18 gauge needles
1	Tevdek 4-0 tie, 24''
2	Prolene 4-0 RB-1 needles
1	Ethilon #2 (D4512)
1	Blood pump bag (for administration of cardioplegia)
1	Peanuts
1	Medium fogarty insert
1	Large lap tape
1	Unvented IV tubing (sterile)
1	30 cc disposable syringe
1	#15 gauge 3'' needle
1	#14 Jelco needle
1	30 cc bottle heparin 1:1000
3	Bowel bags
1	Tevdek 2-0 tie, 24''
1	Umbilical tape
2	Bone wax
1	#13 light cutting needle
1	20 gauge needle
1	10, 15, and 11 knife blades
1	White garbage liner to hold all used instruments

Evaluation in the Intensive Care Unit and Preparation for Surgery

Upon their arrival at the donor hospital, the scrub nurse and anesthesiologist go to the operating room. The scrub nurse begins to set up for the case and checks on the availability of 10–12 liters of chilled saline in pour bottles, while the anesthesiologist checks the anesthesia and monitoring equipment to be used for the cardiectomy. Meanwhile, in the ICU the surgeon examines the donor, with specific attention to heart sounds, breath sounds, and peripheral pulses. If the donor suffered trauma to the body, the chest and back are examined for bruises.

The donor's medical records are thoroughly reviewed at this time. Appropriate notes declaring brain death (two notes are required in California) must be included in the records, as well as consent from legal next-of-kin listing the heart for donation, and notation from the coroner releasing the case for organ recovery. The hemodynamic course of the donor, use of vasopressor agents, 12-lead ECG, echocardiogram, and chest film are examined. Even though these data have been given to the transplant coordinator before the team travels to the donor hospital, the information is always confirmed by the surgeon. The last critical document to be reviewed is a hard copy report of the donor's blood type. Copies of all the records are eventually filed at Stanford. After this information has been thoroughly reviewed, a call is made to the transplant team at Stanford to report the information and to relay any concerns, such as increased dopamine support or deteriorating blood gases. A time estimate is given for returning with the donor heart, and the donor coordinator then makes later follow-up calls.

While the surgeons review the chart, the donor coordinator draws blood samples for tissue typing and lymphocyte cross-match, which will be performed retrospectively at Stanford. The anesthesiologist joins the team in the ICU and inserts a CVP line, arterial line, and volume line if these are not already in place. Before the operation, a recent serum potassium, hematocrit, and arterial blood gas are checked. Four units of blood should be available if needed.

Cardiectomy

Upon arrival in the operating room, the donor coordinator locates the chilled saline, packs it in kick buckets of ice, and places it in the operating room. Since several organs will be recovered from most donors, it is important that the various teams coordinate their techniques before the operation.

During organ recovery, the anesthesiologist is responsible for ade-

quate ventilation, monitoring CVP, blood pressure, heart rate, ECG trac-
ing, temperature, and urine output. Mean arterial pressure should be maintained between 60–80 mmHg. Cardioactive and vasoactive drugs, such as
dopamine and metaraminol, are titrated to the lowest effective doses. The
CVP is maintained between 8–12 mmHg. Blood is generally given to maintain the hematocrit above 30%. An arterial blood gas, potassium, and hematocrit are sent at the start of the case. An oxygen saturation monitor is used
throughout the procedure.

The cardiectomy begins with a median sternotomy. The heart is examined for evidence of contusion, coronary artery disease, recent ischemic
events, valvular heart disease, congenital anomalies, and overall right and
left ventricular contractility. The surgeon then relays these findings to the
donor coordinator along with an estimate of the time needed by the other
recovery teams to complete their dissection. The coordinator reports these
findings to the transplant team at Stanford and the time estimate for returning with the heart. Any important changes in time of return will be com-
municated to Stanford to assure coordination with the recipient operation.

The cardiectomy continues with dissection of the aorta from the pulmonary trunk using electrocautery (Figure 1). The ascending aorta is dissected circumferentially and surrounded with an umbilical tape. The pericardial reflection is incised over the superior vena cava (SVC) to its superior
edge. The SVC is dissected circumferentially for a distance of 2 cm below
the azygos vein. Special care is taken not to injure the sinoatrial node at the
junction of the right atrium with the SVC. The SVC is surrounded with two
free ties so that the length is adequate to cut between them when the heart
is removed. Next, the inferior vena cava (IVC) is cleared circumferentially
from the pericardial reflection and surrounded with an umbilical tape.

When the surgeons recovering additional organs have completed their
dissection, 30,000 units of heparin are given through the SVC. The cardioplegia line is flushed with cardioplegia solution to remove all air bubbles
and connected to a shortened #14 angiocath, which is inserted into the ascending aorta. When all teams are ready, the SVC is tied and cut, and the
IVC is occluded with a Potts clamp and transected. The heart is allowed to
beat until empty, usually 3–4 beats. The aorta is then cross-clamped, and
the cardioplegia is started using a pressurized blood pump. The time of
cross-clamp is noted and relayed to the other transplant teams. Topical
cooling is begun using a total of 8–10 liters of cold saline poured repeatedly
to submerge the heart.

Once the cardioplegia is completed and the heart is cold, the cardioplegia line is removed, and the pericardial well is emptied of cold saline solution. The heart is excised by retracting upward and transecting the right
and left pulmonary veins at the pericardial reflection (Figure 2) then, tran-

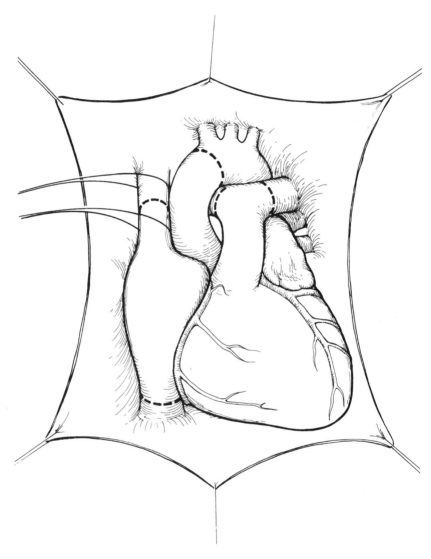

Figure 1. Anticipated lines of transection of the great vessels. The right pulmonary artery may be divided at its origin, or at the pericardial reflection (if there is no combined recovery for lung transplantation).

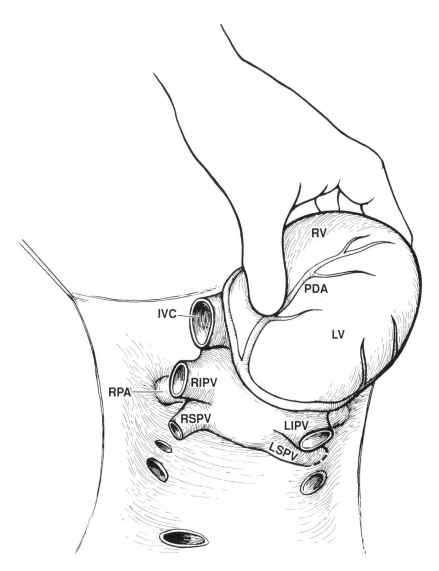

Figure 2. Excision of the donor heart usually begins inferiorly (IVC and pulmonary veins) and proceeds superiorly before transecting the pulmonary arteries and aorta. IVC = inferior vena cava; PV = pulmonary veins (R = right; L = left; I = inferior; S = superior); RPA = right pulmonary artery; RV = right ventricle; LV = left ventricle; PDA = posterior descending artery.

secting the ascending aorta just proximal to the cross-clamp and both pulmonary arteries at the pericardial reflections. If necessary, the ascending aorta can be occluded with the surgeon's left hand, the aortic cross-clamp released and the aorta transected at the arch vessels (for increased length).

Packing and Transporting the Heart

After removal, the heart is rinsed in several basins of cold saline in order to remove blood and to complete endocardial cooling. A sterile bowel bag is opened, and the heart is placed inside with enough cold saline to completely cover it. All air is evacuated as the bag is twisted closed and a tie is placed around it. This bag is placed inside a second bowel bag which is filled with more cold saline and closed similarly. A sterile plastic container is filled with cold saline, and the double-bagged heart is submerged. The canister is sealed and placed in a third bowel bag, which is filled with more cold saline. Air is again evacuated, and the bag is closed by twisting the plastic and tying it off. The canister is then buried in ice in the igloo. This technique results in intramyocardial temperatures, measured in the interventricular septum, in the range of 1°–2°C after 2–3 hours of storage.

After a note is written in the donor's chart briefly describing the procedure and findings, the donor transport team returns to Stanford. Depending on the distance to be traveled, an additional call may be made en route to update the recipient team of the expected time of arrival. A final alert is always given when the team is approximately 10 minutes from the hospital.

Upon arrival in the operating room at Stanford, the donor surgeon will stand by to open the canister when the recipient surgeon is ready. At this time, any relevant information about the excision of the heart is relayed to the implanting team. The donor cross-clamp time is given to the anesthesiologist for notation on the recipient's chart.

Appendix

Abbreviations

Anti-HBc = total antibody to hepatitis B core antigen
Anti-HBs = antibody to hepatitis B surface antigen
Anti-HIV = antibody to human immunodeficiency virus
BP = blood pressure

CMV = cytomegalovirus
CNS = central nervous system
CVP = central venous pressure
DDAVP = desmopressin acetate
$F_i O_2$ = fraction of inspired oxygen
HBsAG = hepatitis B surface antigen
ICU = intensive care unit
IV = intravenous
IVC = inferior vena cava
OR = operating room
PA = pulmonary artery
PDA = posterior descending artery
PEEP = positive end-expiratory pressure
PO_2 = oxygen partial pressure
PV = pulmonary vein (R = right; L = left; I = inferior; S = superior)
SA = sinoatrial
SVC = superior vena cava
UNOS = United Network for Organ Sharing

Selected References

1. Emery RW, Cork RC, Levinson MM, et al. The cardiac donor: A six-year experience. Ann Thorac Surg 1986;41:365–372.
2. Evans RW, Manninen DL, Garrison LP Jr, et al. Donor availability as the primary determinant of the future of heart transplantation. JAMA 1986;255:1892–1898.
3. Fentz V, Gornsen J. Electrocardiographic patterns in patients with cerebrovascular accidents. Circulation 1962;25:22.
4. Gilbert EM, Krueger SK, Murray JL, et al. Echocardiographic evaluation of potential cardiac transplant donors. J Thorac Cardiovasc Surg 1988;95:1003–1007.
5. Griepp RB, Stinson EB, Clark DA, et al. The cardiac donor. Surg Gynecol Obstet 1971;133:792–798.
6. Lower RR, Shumway NE. Studies on the orthotopic homotransplantation of the canine heart. Surg Forum 1960;11:18.
7. McManus RP, O'Hair DP, Beitzinger JM, et al. Patients who die awaiting heart transplantation. J Heart Lung Transplant 1993;12:159–172.
8. Novitzky D, Cooper DK, Zuhdi N. Triiodothyronine therapy in the cardiac transplant recipient. Transplant Proc 1988;20:65–68.
9. Report of the medical consultants on the diagnoses of death to the President's Commission for the Study of Ethical Problems in Medicine. JAMA 1981;246: 2184–2186.
10. Webb WR, Howard HS. Restoration of function of the refrigerated heart. Surg Forum 1957;8:313.
11. Yacoub M, Mankad P, Ledingham S. Donor procurement and surgical techniques for cardiac transplantation. Semin Thorac Cardiovasc Surg 1990;2: 153–161.

Chapter 3

Cardiac Transplant Admission, Anesthesia, and Operative Procedures

Patrick M. McCarthy, M.D.,
Julian A. Smith, M.B., M.S., FRACS,
Lawrence C. Siegel, M.D., Ray H. Engstrom, M.D.,
David C. Fitzgerald, M.D., George E. Sarris, M.D.,
Edward B. Stinson, M.D.

Several months usually elapse from the transplant recipient's initial evaluation until a donor heart becomes available. The hospital admission, just hours before the transplant operation, is an important time to reevaluate and prepare the recipient. Much has to be done by the nursing, surgery, and anesthesia staff, and an organized system of procedures is necessary.

Preadmission

Notifying the Patient

The patient is notified by telephone that a potential donor is being evaluated and is closely questioned about any changes in physical status, especially any recent infections. The patient's overall status (e.g., change in peripheral edema, worsening dyspnea, ascites, etc.) and any other recent illnesses are also evaluated. During this telephone call, the patient is also instructed not to eat or drink anything (except medications), to stay near a telephone, and to make arrangements with family or work as needed.

At the same time, the transplant cardiologist who evaluated and follows the recipient is contacted to review the details of the case and discuss any

From: Smith JA, McCarthy PM, Sarris GE, Stinson EB, Reitz BA (eds.): The Stanford Manual of Cardiopulmonary Transplantation. Futura Publishing Co., Inc., Armonk, NY, 1996.

Table 1
Timing the Procedures of the Recipient and Donor Teams

Recipient Team	Donor Team
Admission	Departure for other hospital
Evaluation	Donor evaluation
To operating room	Anticipated 1-1/2 hours until return
Anesthesia induced	Donor heart inspected and judged acceptable
Skin incision	Anticipated 30 minutes until return
Recipient cannulated	Donor heart arrives

recent changes that might create problems perioperatively. If there are concerns that the recipient has developed an infection or other illness that may prevent an operation at this time, another recipient should be alerted to be on standby.

Transporting and Admitting the Recipient

When the surgeon has gathered enough information on the donor and verified that the recipient is in satisfactory condition, then arrangements should be made to admit the recipient. It is important to bring the recipient into the hospital as quickly as possible so that there is plenty of time for preoperative preparation. Transport is usually by car with family, but it may require helicopter, fixed-wing, or prearranged jet aircraft. Notification also must be given to admissions, the admitting floor, the operating room, the anesthesiologist, and the postoperative intensive care unit (ICU). Usually, the donor team is simultaneously being transported to the donor hospital and will be working quickly with other organ procurement groups to return the donor organs (Table 1).

Admission Procedures

Admission to the Floor

The patient is usually sent from admissions to radiology to have posterior-anterior and lateral chest films taken. The patient and chest films are then sent directly to the admitting floor. The time spent on the admitting floor varies from a few minutes to several hours depending on the timing with the return of the donor team.

The nursing staff admits the patient, obtains vital signs and weight, then reviews the consent forms with the patient and family. Blood is drawn and sent for type and cross-match (four units packed red blood cells and four units whole blood, all cytomegalovirus [CMV] negative for CMV negative recipients) and for stat lab work (complete blood count, platelet count, electrolytes, renal and hepatic panel, and prothrombin time). A urinalysis is also sent. If time permits, a large bore peripheral intravenous (IV) line is placed and kept open with a normal saline infusion.

Physician Evaluation

Before the recipient is sent to the operating room, the following points should be covered:

History and examination
Chest film
Basic lab work
Type and cross-match (verify blood type)
Fresh frozen plasma and vitamin K
Azathioprine (4 mg/kg) IV
No preoperative cyclosporine is given

The admitting resident obtains a rapid but thorough history and physical examination. Like the initial telephone conversation, these procedures should emphasize any recent infections or change in physical status. Deterioration of the patient's physical condition should be noted, specifically hepatomegaly, ascites, peripheral edema, and lung changes from pulmonary edema or pleural effusions. The chest film should also be examined for evidence of infection, pulmonary edema, or effusions.

At this point, the physician should reassure the patient and his/her family because they will understandably be anxious. This is an excellent opportunity to review the forthcoming procedures and explain what the patient and family should expect in the early phase. Questions are answered and the consent forms reviewed. This is time well spent, as the doctor-patient relationship is unusually close with transplant patients and their families.

If possible, the results of the blood work should be reviewed before the patient is sent to the operating room. Additionally, the patient's blood type should be reconfirmed with the blood bank to avoid the disaster that would happen if a clerical error had been made when the recipient's blood type was recorded. Most of these patients are receiving warfarin, and two units of fresh frozen plasma may be given intravenously, often with 20 mg of phytonadione (Aquamephyton) intramuscularly. Alternatively, in the case of primary sternotomy, fresh frozen plasma may simply be added to the pump prime. Finally, azathioprine (4 mg/kg) is given intravenously. Preoperative cyclosporine is not used. The immunosuppression regimen is discussed further in Chapter 6.

Anesthetic Management of the Heart Transplant Recipient

Preoperative Anesthetic Evaluation and Premedication

The standard preanesthetic evaluation should be supplemented with considerations particular to these patients. Since progression of cardiovascular disease is usually well documented, a history of recent exacerbation of cardiac dysfunction should be sought, and cardiac catheterization data should be interpreted in light of interval changes. The patient may have a history of ventricular dysrhythmia, and the effectiveness of past antidysrhythmic therapy should be reviewed. Catheterization may also reveal the presence of pulmonary hypertension and elevated pulmonary vascular resistance (PVR). If this is the case, severity of the abnormality and responsiveness to specific vasodilators must be determined. The patient's history, physical examination, and laboratory studies are used to find evidence of renal and hepatic dysfunction. The medication schedule should be verified, particular attention paid to the recent use of inotropes, diuretics, antidysrhythmics, anticoagulants, immunosuppressive agents, and noncardiovascular medications.

Although anxious, these patients are usually well informed and psychologically prepared. They respond well to the reassurance of the preoperative visit, and pharmacologic premedication is usually not necessary. Reassuring the family of patients who have rapidly progressive cardiac dysfunction is valuable. Oxygen therapy should be started before the patient is transported to the operative suite.

Anesthetic Equipment, Monitoring, and Vascular Access

When the patient arrives in the operative suite, he/she should be placed on the operating table, and oxygen and noninvasive monitors should be applied. Dyspnea in the supine position may be treated by raising the back of the operating table. Noninvasive monitors include:

Pulse oximetry
Five-lead electrocardiography with ST segment analysis. Leads should

be covered with tape to ensure that electrical contact is not degraded by prep solution or blood.

Automated blood pressure measurement

Precordial stethoscope

Aseptic technique is important, as infection is a much feared complication in the immunosuppressed transplant patient. Airway equipment is presterilized with a disposable circle system and bacterial filters. In addition, aseptic technique is used in inserting and securing all vascular catheters.

A 14- or 16-gauge IV catheter is inserted. Midazolam (0.5 mg) or fentanyl (50 ug) may be titrated intravenously to assure patient comfort. A second IV catheter is inserted in patients who have had a previous sternotomy. A 20-gauge catheter is placed percutaneously in a radial artery. A central venous catheter is usually inserted before anesthesia is induced. If the patient is very dyspneic in the supine position, or if the initial time estimate for the arrival of the graft is substantially in error, it may be advantageous to insert the central venous catheter following anesthetic induction. A triple lumen catheter is used for patients who do not have significant pulmonary hypertension, but for patients with elevated PVR an 8.5 Fr introducer is used since a pulmonary artery catheter may be necessary to manage right heart failure after transplantation. The left internal jugular vein is the preferred site of cannulation, so that the right internal jugular vein remains unscarred for repeated endomyocardial biopsies of the transplanted heart.

Anesthetic Induction and Maintenance

Anesthesia is not induced until the team harvesting the graft reports that the donor heart appears to be normal to direct inspection (Table 1). The patient is preoxygenated with 100% oxygen. Continuous airway gas analysis should be used. The patient is at risk for pulmonary aspiration of gastric contents because of the unscheduled nature of the operation. Cricoid pressure must be used.

The following induction agents are used:

Fentanyl (5–20 ug/kg) or sufentanil (1–4 ug/kg)

Etomidate (0.1–0.2 mg/kg) is useful for permitting rapid airway control and for assuring the lack of patient awareness. Midazolam may also be used.

Vecuronium (0.15 mg/kg), pancuronium (0.1 mg/kg), or a combination of these agents should be administered immediately to permit airway control. Hypercarbia and hypoxemia must be avoided; thus immediate control of the airway is crucial. Narcotic-induced chest wall rigidity must be prevented.

The patient can be expected to have a low cardiac output. The speed of induction can be significantly delayed. This delay must be anticipated to avoid overdosage. The low cardiac output and volume-contracted condition make the patient unusually sensitive to anesthetics initially. A high preload may be necessary, and IV fluid is often administered to compensate for the vasodilating effect of anesthetic-mediated sympatholysis. If induction is poorly tolerated, the patient may require inotropic support.

The patient should be ventilated by mask, and cricoid pressure should be released only after the airway has been secured with a cuffed endotracheal tube. The usual aids for managing the unexpectedly difficult airway should be readily available. Antibiotics are administered. The following additional monitors are inserted:

Urinary catheter with thermistor
Nasopharyngeal temperature probe
Esophageal stethoscope

If the anticipated arrival of the graft is delayed, the donor should be covered and kept warm and the skin preparation should be delayed. Additional narcotics should be administered only when surgery is about to begin.

Although the patient's low cardiac output and volume-contracted condition make the patient unusually sensitive to anesthetics during induction, the volume of distribution of anesthetics will be fairly normal. Typical cumulative doses are as follows:

Fentanyl, 50 ug/kg, or sufentanil 10–15 ug/kg
Midazolam, 0.2 mg/kg
Vecuronium, 0.3 mg/kg or pancuronium, 0.2 mg/kg
Scopolamine, 0.07 mg/kg

The Heart Transplant Operation

Timing and Opening

Ideally, the recipient should be in the operating room and cannulated for cardiopulmonary bypass (CPB) when the heart returns. To allow adequate time for anesthesia, prepping, opening, and cannulation, we usually send the recipient to the operating room about 1-1/2 hours before the expected return of the donor team (Table 1). The skin incision is planned for approximately 30 minutes before the anticipated arrival of the donor team.

The patient is positioned supine on the operating table with both arms tucked in at the side. The patient is prepped from neck to knees and draped so that the whole groin area is accessible. A standard median sternotomy is made. The pericardium is opened in the midline, reflected laterally, and suspended. The heart is typically very enlarged, which may make exposure and cannulation difficult. The heart may be especially irritable and prone to arrhythmias, resulting in hypotension or fibrillation during sternotomy and cannulation. In the presence of adhesions due to previous cardiac surgery, only enough dissection should be performed to expose the aortic and atrial cannulation sites. The remaining dissection should be performed only after cannulation and decompression of the heart. The heart should be disturbed as little as possible, and the surgical team should be experienced enough to cannulate rapidly if the patient's hemodynamics deteriorate.

Cannulation

Standard cannulation after heparinization includes an arterial cannula in the ascending aorta just below the innominate artery and two caval cannulas: a right angle cannula and the inferior vena cava (IVC) cannula. The right angle cannula is positioned in the superior vena cava (SVC). The cannula can be inserted close to the recipient sinoatrial (SA) node because injury to the node has no significant consequence. The IVC cannula is inserted in the right atrium just superior to its juncture with the IVC. If necessary to make placement easier, the inferior cannula can be placed after CPB has decompressed the heart. Both cannulas should be placed far lateral in the right atrium to allow an adequate atrial cuff when the recipient's heart is excised. Tapes are passed around the SVC and IVC. If the timing with the donor team has been well coordinated, it should be only a short wait until the donor heart arrives.

Cardiectomy

When the donor team arrives, CPB is established, and the patient is cooled to 28°C. The caval tapes are snared. The recipient's heart is excised when the donor team is in the operating room. The aortic cross-clamp is applied. The right atrium is opened at the base of the atrial appendage (Figure 1). The incision is extended inferiorly, staying close to the atrioventricular (AV) groove, with care taken to leave a 5 to 10 mm atrial cuff along the IVC cannula. The incision is brought down to the lateral side of the coronary sinus, and then brought superiorly around the atrial appendage to the septum between right and left atrium. Next, the aorta is transected just above the aortic valve, taking care not to injure the right pulmonary

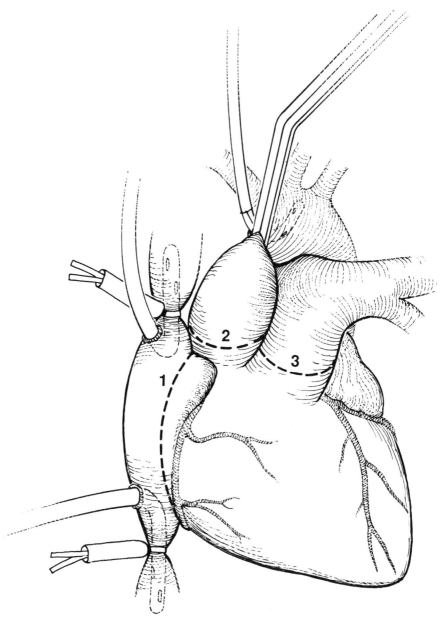

Figure 1. Cannulation for transplant. Dashed lines show incisions for cardiectomy: 1 = right atrial incision; 2 = aorta transected at level of commissures; 3 = pulmonary artery transected at level of pulmonary valve; left atrial and atrial septum incisions not shown.

artery behind the aorta. Next, the pulmonary artery is transected, being careful to stay close to the pulmonary valve, and not to bevel the posterior wall of the pulmonary artery. Finally, the heart is pulled superiorly and to the left, and the left atrium is divided starting at the septum and extending across the dome to the base of the left atrial appendage. The incision is continued inferiorly close to the mitral valve.

The heart is removed when the left atrial incision reaches the right atrial incision at the coronary sinus. The surgeon should cauterize bleeding points in the connective tissue along the cut edge of the left atrium and between the aorta and pulmonary artery. In addition, palpation or suction within the main and branch pulmonary arteries at this point will allow the surgeon to remove pulmonary emboli that were not suspected preoperatively.

Donor Heart Preparation

The donor heart is removed from the ice chest, and the outermost plastic bag is opened with scissors. The sterile inner bag is carefully removed from the transport canister and placed into a sterile basin. The bag is opened and the heart is removed, and placed into another basin with cold sterile saline and brought to the operating field.

The epicardial fat may solidify, especially with a long preservation time, but the fat will quickly thaw in the cold saline. First, the pulmonary artery and aorta are separated to a level approximately 1 cm above the left main coronary artery. Next, the plane between the pulmonary artery and left atrium (the transverse sinus) is found, and the connective tissues are divided. The pulmonary artery is transected at its bifurcation. The heart is then turned over, and the four pulmonary veins are identified and opened. The posterior left atrial wall is opened, and the irregular ends of the pulmonary veins are trimmed away.

It is important to look for a patent foramen ovale (PFO) in both the donor and recipient because early posttransplant hypoxemia may occur if right heart pressures are elevated. If a PFO is identified, it should be closed from the right atrial side. The donor mitral and aortic valves are also inspected for congenital or acquired abnormalities because of their potential importance to the patient's long-term management.

Atrial Anastomoses

The atrial anastomoses are performed with a 54-inch, 3–0 polypropylene suture. The first stitch is placed in the recipient left atrium at the level of the left superior pulmonary vein (Figure 2). The ends of the suture are brought through until an equal length on either side is reached, and the end outside the recipient left atrium is tagged to the drapes. The assistant holds the donor heart near the left side of the chest with the left atrium turned superiorly. The stitch is then passed from inside out through the donor left atrium at the level of the left atrial appendage. The donor heart is lowered into the pericardium, and the donor left atrium is exposed. The inferior left atrial suture line is then anastomosed with a continuous suture (Figure 3). The residual coronary sinus wall of the recipient should be incorporated into the suture line. When the atrial septum is reached inferiorly, the suture is tagged outside the donor left atrium. The other end of the suture is then used to close the superior left atrium and atrial septum. The assistant retracts the donor great vessels inferiorly to expose this area. Size discrepancy should be made up gradually, but a large discrepancy can easily be accommodated, especially along the septum. The ends of the suture are tied outside the left atrium. While the superior aspect of the left atrium is being sutured, the

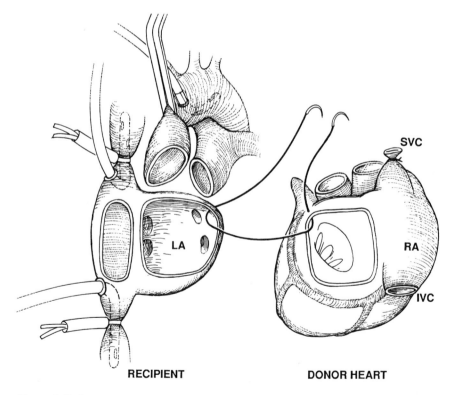

RECIPIENT   **DONOR HEART**

Figure 2. Left atrial anastomosis starts by lining up the left superior pulmonary vein (recipient) and left atrial appendage (donor). LA = left atrium; SVC = superior vena cava; RA = right ventricle; IVC = inferior vena cava.

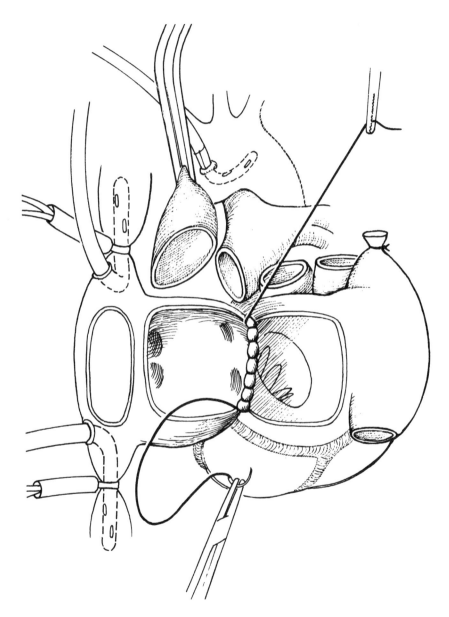

Figure 3. Left atrial anastomosis proceeds along the inferior wall above the left pulmonary veins.

artery to the donor sinus node will occasionally be near the suture line, and it should be identified and avoided. Direct trauma (as with forceps) to the donor sinus node should be avoided during exposure and suturing.

When the left atrial suture line is completed, a slow infusion of cold saline (3°–4°C) is started into the pericardial well, and is continuously removed by low power suction. Also, the left atrial appendage is cannulated with another line of cold saline (not shown in the illustrations) for continuous endocardial cooling and evacuation of air from the left heart. In other transplant programs, cardioplegia is given to the donor heart to maintain cardiac cooling and arrest.

Next, the donor right atrium is opened. The incision is started on the lateral aspect of the IVC and extends up to the base of the right atrial ap-

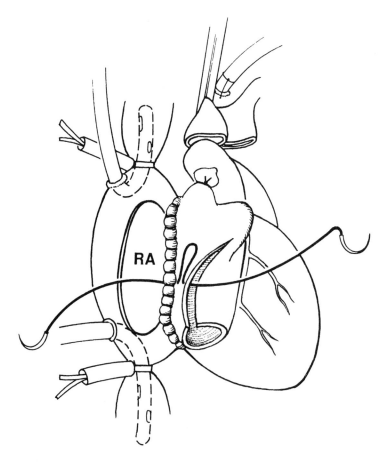

Figure 4. Donor right atrium has been opened from the IVC to the base of the right atrial appendage. Anastomosis is started along the atrial septum. RA = right atrium.

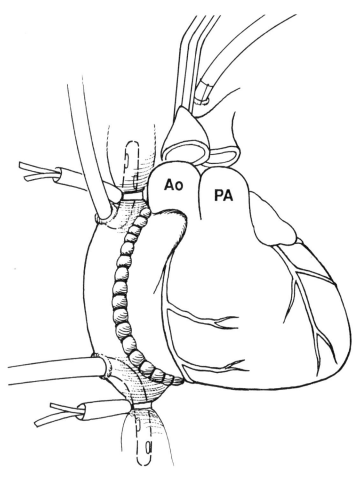

Figure 5. Atrial anastomoses have been completed. The great vessels are aligned and trimmed appropriately. Rewarming on bypass is started. Ao = aorta; PA = pulmonary artery.

pendage (Figure 4). The first stitch is placed in the midportion of the donor right atrium and then passed through the midportion of the suture line along the atrial septum. The bites along the septum have to be taken deeply, and care should be taken to smooth out the ridge along the right atrial suture line so that a bioptome will be able to cross it easily. The right atrial suture line is first brought inferiorly and tagged when the suture is advanced beyond the IVC cannula. The other end of the stitch is then brought superiorly to complete the anastomosis (Figure 5). Systemic rewarming is started when the right atrial anastomosis is complete.

Great Vessel Anastomoses

The proper length of the donor pulmonary artery should be determined and trimmed. If it is too long, torsion and kinking may occur. The pulmonary artery anastomosis is performed with running 4–0 polypropylene. First, the back wall is sutured starting at the left lateral side of the recipient pulmonary artery (Figure 6); then the anterior wall is completed using the other end of the suture. Care should be taken to orient the pul-

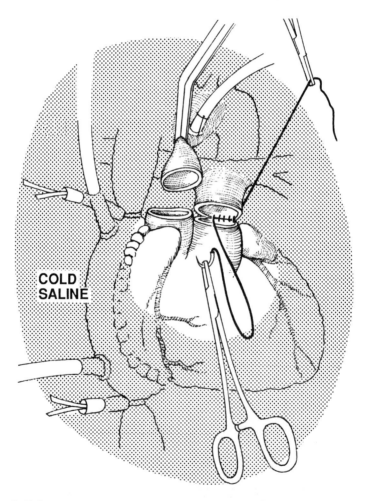

Figure 6. Pulmonary artery is anastomosed while the heart is immersed in cold saline (shaded area) for continuous topical cooling. Posterior wall is sewn first.

monary artery properly and marking sutures may help with this orientation. Avoid pursestringing the anastomosis while following the suture or tying. We used to perform the aortic anastomosis before the pulmonary artery anastomosis to decrease the graft ischemic time. However, the few extra minutes of ischemic time are generally an acceptable tradeoff to be able to perform the pulmonary artery anastomosis in a bloodless field and

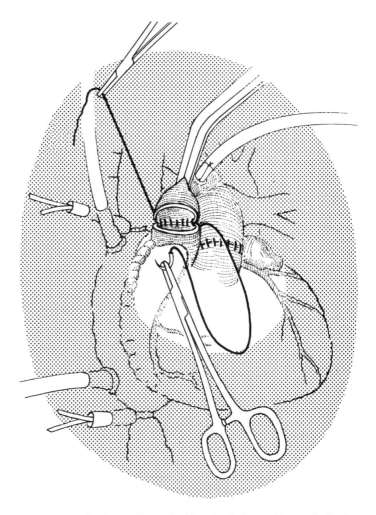

Figure 7. Aortic anastomosis is also performed with a single layer. Alternatively, the aortic anastomosis may be performed before the pulmonary artery anastomosis, so that the aortic cross-clamp is removed and the pulmonary artery sewn while the heart is perfused and beating.

to allow more effective deairing of the graft by transient filling of the right heart.

Finally, the aortic anastomosis is performed with running 4–0 polypropylene (Figure 7). The anastomosis is performed in the same way as the pulmonary artery anastomosis, with the same potential problems. If the donor aorta is small, discrepancies in size may be compensated for by opening the donor aorta anteriorly for 1–2 cm.

Completing the Operation

To complete the operation, the caval tapes are removed, the head of the bed is lowered, and the infusions of cold saline are stopped. An air vent is placed on the donor aorta, or the cardioplegia administration site is used to vent the aorta. Blood is transfused to fill the heart while the lungs are intermittently inflated. The cross-clamp is removed, and deairing procedures are continued as needed. Removal of the cross-clamp marks the end of the graft ischemic time and should be noted by the anesthesiologist. The left atrial appendage line is removed, and the hole oversewn. Most hearts will defibrillate spontaneously. Temporary ventricular and atrial (on the *donor* atrium) pacing wires are always placed. Suture lines are checked for bleed-

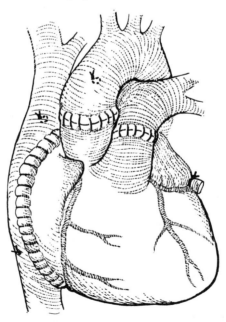

Figure 8. Completed operation after decannulation.

ing. After approximately 30 minutes of reperfusion of the transplanted heart and restoration of adequate cardiac contraction and rhythm, CPB is weaned and the cannulas are removed (Figure 8).

Termination of Cardiopulmonary Bypass

Junctional rhythm is common in the denervated transplanted heart immediately after resuscitation. Isoproterenol (10–75 ng/kg per min) titrated to produce a heart rate of 90–120 beats/minute optimizes cardiac output, which is rate dependent in the early postoperative period. When sinus rhythm is achieved, two P waves are commonly observed. The residual recipient atrial tissue produces nonconducting P waves. Responses mediated by vagal tone will be observed in the rate of the recipient atrium, but they have no clinical importance beyond the ease with which the electrocardiogram (ECG) can be interpreted. Atropine and neostigmine do not affect the donor heart rate. Hypertension does not produce reflex bradycardia. The graft atrium produces normally conducted P waves. The graft conductive tissue contains adrenergic receptors and responds in an appropriate manner to norepinephrine, epinephrine, and isoproterenol.

Inotropic support with dopamine and epinephrine may be necessary, especially if an abnormal pulmonary circulation causes right ventricular failure. Sodium nitroprusside is used to reduce the afterload and prostaglandin E_1 (PGE_1) (20–100 ng/kg per min) and nitroglycerin may be used for additional pulmonary vasodilation, especially if a preoperative catheterization study demonstrated responsiveness of the pulmonary circulation. IV fluid and vasodilators must be given with particular care, as the flow produced by the denervated heart is quite sensitive to preload.

Post-bypass bleeding is a common problem brought on by the preoperative use of anticoagulants, the depressed synthetic function of the liver in chronic heart failure, and the trauma of CPB. After administration of protamine, infusion of platelets, fresh frozen plasma, and red blood cells may be necessary. Cryoprecipitate may also occasionally be needed, especially for patients undergoing repeat sternotomy. There may be little urine production, especially if the patient has received high dose diuretics preoperatively. Mannitol and furosemide may be needed to induce diuresis. Methylprednisolone (500 mg) is given intravenously after CPB has been discontinued.

If the pleural spaces have been opened, or if there are pleural effusions (frequently these are present), they are drained with separate pleural chest tubes. The chest is closed in the usual fashion, and extra care should be taken to obtain a secure sternal closure.

The patient is then transferred directly to the ICU using a sterile, disposable Jackson-Rees system.

Bicaval Anastomotic Technique

Recently we have used a modification of this conventional Stanford technique for orthotopic cardiac transplantation (Figures 9–11). The donor left atrium is sewn to a recipient pulmonary venous cuff and separate SVC and IVC anastomoses are substituted for the single right atrial anastomosis.

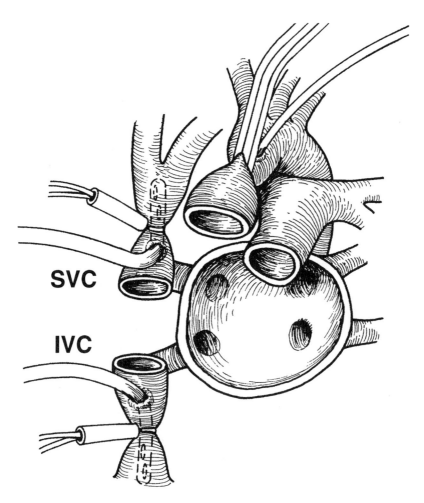

Figure 9. Appearance following recipient cardiectomy for bicaval anastomotic technique. Superior vena caval (SVC) and inferior vena caval (IVC) cuffs instead of a right atrial cuff.

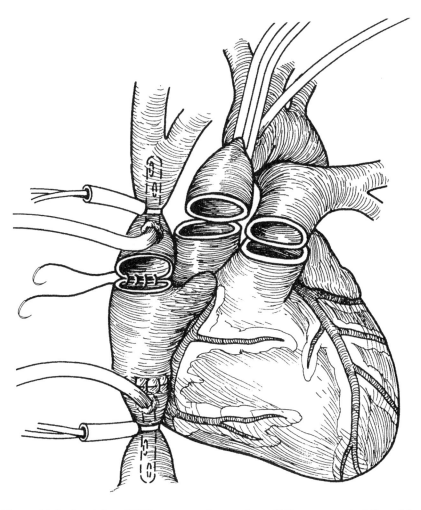

Figure 10. Left atrial and IVC anastomosis complete. SVC anastomosis followed by pulmonary arterial and aortic anastomoses.

The advantages of this technique are the maintenance of atrial shape, the preservation of sinus node function, and improved AV valvular competence. Separate caval anastomoses are useful in situations of large discrepancies between the donor and recipient right atrium. The technique is valuable in transplants performed for congenital heart disease and we have also used bicaval anastomoses for heart-lung transplantation (see Chapter 10). An aesthetically pleasing appearance of the implanted heart is noted at the completion of the transplant.

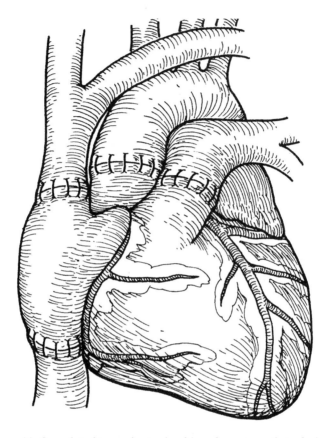

Figure 11. Completed transplant using bicaval anastomotic technique.

Special Circumstances

Reoperations

Many patients require a resternotomy because of previous coronary artery bypass, valve replacement, or transplant. The early phases of the operation are carried out in the usual careful fashion required by these cases. Tissue planes, especially if the lung was exposed at the earlier operation, need to be carefully followed to avoid bleeding problems or air leaks. Usually, the recipient aorta is excised along with any proximal bypass graft anastomoses, or, with a short aorta, the proximal anastomoses are left in place and oversewn. When the start time is coordinated with the anticipated arrival of the donor team, additional time should be allowed for the dissection and cannulation (about 60 minutes starting from skin incision).

Implantable Cardioverter-Defibrillators and Pacemakers

Implantable cardioverter-defibrillators (ICDs) should be deactivated using a magnet before the patient is prepped. Dissection around the electrode patches is frequently difficult if they are closely related to the left phrenic nerve; often, a posterior patch is left in place if it is extrapericardial. However, if at all possible, all foreign material should be removed to avoid the possibility of later infection. Intrapericardial ICD patches may create an intense inflammatory reaction that complicates and slows the cannulation process. The generator and lead remnants are removed after the sternum has been closed.

Pacemakers are handled in the same way as an ordinary cardiac case, either by avoiding cautery until the heart is exposed or by using a magnet to place the pacemaker in a backup mode. The pacemaker generator and divided leads are removed at the end of the operation.

Heterotopic Cardiac Transplantation

Heterotopic (piggyback) transplants have been performed only twice at Stanford. For patients with cardiomyopathy and elevated, fixed PVR, heart-lung transplantation is recommended.

Pediatric Heart Transplantation

Anesthetic Management

The pathophysiology of the pediatric heart transplant candidate can be divided into two groups:

1. those with single ventricle physiology (e.g., hypoplastic left ventricle); and
2. those with low output states secondary to ventricular failure (e.g., cardiomyopathy, endocardial fibroelastosis, and anomalous coronary artery).

Single Ventricle Physiology

In this condition, systemic and pulmonary circulations are in parallel. Ductal patency and interatrial communication are usually required for mixing between the two circulations to occur. For each ventricular contraction, the amount of the stroke volume delivered to the pulmonary and systemic beds depends on the balance between the systemic vascular resistance and PVR. In this age group, PVR is very responsive to metabolic manipulations (Table 2).

In general, patients maintain an oxygen saturation of 80%–90% and mean arterial pressures of 45–65 mmHg. They are often on PGE_1 infusions to maintain ductal patency and have a PFO or a Rashkind atrial septostomy to ensure adequate pulmonary venous drainage. They are often intubated either secondary to PGE_1-induced apnea or for better control of ventilation and PVR. Rarely, low dose dopamine is required secondary to mild ventricular failure.

Low Output States

This condition in children is similar to the condition of adults who present for heart transplantation with cardiac failure. Cardiac output is highly dependent on rate since stroke volume is nearly fixed. Small increases in afterload will significantly decrease cardiac output. The Frank-Starling curve is lower and flattened, but maximum filling pressures must still be maintained to optimize already marginal cardiac output. Myocardium shows down regulation of beta-adrenergic receptors; therefore, patients may require higher than normal levels of inotropic drugs. There may be varying

Table 2
Metabolic Manipulations of Pulmonary Vascular Resistance

Increased PVR	Decreased PVR
Low F_iO_2	High F_iO_2
High $PaCO_2$	Low $PaCO_2$ (alkalosis)
High or low lung volumes	Lung volume at FRC
High airway pressure	Beta$_2$ agonists (Isuprel)
High hematocrit (>50%)	Pulmonary vasodilators (PGE_1, NTG, tolazoline)
Pressors (alpha-agonists)	Anesthesia
Hypothermia	

FRC = functional residual capacity; NTG = Nitroglycerine; PVR = pulmonary vasculature resistance.

Table 3
Drugs and Drips for Pediatric Heart Transplantation

Drugs to be Drawn Up and Labeled

Drug	Concentration	Type of Syringe	Dosage
Fentanyl	50 ug/cc	5 cc	titrated
Midazolam	1 mg/cc	10 cc	titrated
Pancuronium	1 mg/cc	10 cc	0.1 mg/kg
Vecuronium	1 mg/cc	10 cc	0.1 mg/kg
Calcium chloride	100 mg/cc	5 cc	20 mg/kg × 3 doses
Sodium bicarbonate	1 meq/cc	5 cc	1.0 meq/kg
Epinephrine	1 ug/cc	3 cc	0.03 ug/kg
Phenylephrine	100 ug/cc	10 cc	(for CPB)
Phenylephrine	10 ug/cc	3 cc	1–5 ug/kg
Atropine	0.5 mg/cc	3 cc	20 ug/kg
Cefamandol	50 mg/cc	10 cc	25 mg/kg
Erythromycin	50 mg/cc	10 cc	10 mg/kg
Phentolamine*	0.5 mg/cc	10 cc	0.2 mg/kg
Methylprednisolone*	50 mg/cc		15 mg/kg pre&post CPB
Furosemide	10 mg/cc		0.5–1.0 mg/kg
Mannitol	250 mg/cc		0.5–1.0 gram/kg
Magnesium sulfate	500 mg/cc		20 mg/kg slow infusion
Potassium chloride**	2 meq/cc		slow IV infusion
DDAVP	4 mcg/cc		0.3 mcg/kg
Amicar	250 mg/cc		100 mg/kg loading
(Epsilon aminocaproic acid)			(20 mg/kg/hr infusion)

Drips Commonly Used

Drug	Preparation	Final Concentration	Dosage
Dopamine	200 mg in 250 cc	800 ug/cc	5–15 ug/kg/min
Nitroglycerine	50 mg in 250 cc	200 ug/cc	0.5–3.0 ug/kg/min
Nitroprusside	50 mg in 250 cc	200 ug/cc	0.5–3.0 ug/kg/min
Epinephrine	2 mg in 250 cc	8 ug/cc	25–250 ng/kg/min
Isoproterenol	2 mg in 250 cc	8 ug/cc	25–250 ng/kg/min
ProstaglandinE$_1$	500 ug in 100 cc	5 ug/cc	25–200 ng/kg/min
Lidocaine	1 gm in 250 cc	4 mg/cc	10–50 ug/kg/min

*Only for circulatory arrest cases.
**KCL dose needed (meq) = (desired serum K - acutal serum K) × weight (kg) × 0.3.
CPB = cardiopulmonary bypass; DDAVP = desmopressin acetate.

degrees of pulmonary edema, fixed and reversible increases in PVR, hepatic dysfunction with coagulopathy, and renal failure.

A heating blanket, anesthesia circuit humidifier, overhead radiant warmer, and increased operating room temperature are used to prevent hypothermia after the bypass operation. Most patients are critically ill and do not require premedication. Monitoring includes ECG, pulse oximeter (multiple probes in case of failure), blood pressure cuff, oral and rectal temperature probes, Foley catheter, end-tidal CO_2, central venous pressure (CVP), and arterial catheter. Table 3 lists the drugs and drips with the dosages used in pediatric heart transplantation.

General Guidelines for Vessel Cannulation

In patients with congenital cardiac disease and intracardiac shunts, we cannot overstress the need to avoid air in intravascular lines. Our current practice is to attempt arterial percutaneous and central venous catheterization on almost all patients. The exceptions are low birth weight neonates with umbilical artery catheters in place or small infants with nonpalpable pulses. If difficulty is encountered achieving arterial cannulation, the radial artery on one side must be left untouched for a cutdown by the surgeons. Central venous access is accomplished in almost all cases via the left internal jugular vein with a 4 Fr double lumen catheter. With experience it can be achieved in more than 90% of cases. The right internal jugular vein is reserved for future cardiac biopsies in older children. If central venous access is unsuccessful, the surgeons will place a transthoracic line at an appropriate time intraoperatively with a 4 Fr double lumen CVP. Transthoracic intracardiac lines are occasionally placed to monitor pulmonary artery, and right atrial or left atrial pressures posttransplantation. A transducer system should be available to transduce these lines after they are passed over the drapes. Because these patients will be immunosuppressed, meticulous aseptic technique must be used.

Induction and Precardiopulmonary Bypass

All patients must be considered to have a full stomach. Induction is a modified rapid sequence with cricoid pressure using fentanyl (30–50 ug/kg) with pancuronium (0.1 mg/kg intravenously). Antibiotics (cefamandole, 25 mg/kg; erythromycin, 10 mg/kg) are also given. In patients with single ventricle physiology, previous ventilatory parameters and F_iO_2 must be maintained after induction. Marked increased F_iO_2 and ventilation can result in increased SaO_2 (95%–100%), hypotension, systemic hypoperfusion, and acidosis. Patients with a chronic low cardiac output state may require abnormally high levels of inotropic support secondary to alpha-adrenergic receptor down regulation. A phosphodiesterase-2 inhibitor (e.g., amrinone) may be added that bypasses the beta-receptor. Also, in these patients, cardiac output is highly dependent on a low afterload (SVR), high heart rate, and adequate preload. Fentanyl (100 ug/kg) is added to the CPB prime to maintain adequate drug levels in the face of CPB dilution. For circulatory arrest (hypoplastic left ventricle), methylprednisolone (15 mg/kg), phenytoin (5.0 mg/kg), phentolamine (0.2 mg/kg), and furosemide (1 mg/kg) are added to CPB prime. To ensure minimal body oxygen consumption, pancuronium (0.2 mg/kg) should be given before cardiac arrest. Ice bags are placed around the head. When CPB is reinstituted, a second dose of phentolamine (0.2 mg/kg) should be given to aid in rewarming.

Postcardiopulmonary Bypass

The transplanted denervated heart retains its intrinsic control mechanisms and responds typically to drugs that act directly on the heart without involvement of autonomic innervation. Examples of such drugs are dopamine, norepinephrine, epinephrine, and isoproterenol. Drugs that exert their cardiac effects through indirect autonomic mechanisms will have no effect on heart rate. Examples include atropine, digoxin, pancuronium, and anticholinesterase. Inotropic support with dopamine (5–10 mcg/kg per min) is frequently required. Less commonly, epinephrine (25–50 ng/kg per min) may be needed. Additional fentanyl is given for signs of inadequate levels of anesthesia (e.g., hypertension and high pulmonary artery pressures). Coagulopathy after bypass is treated with infusion of CMV negative fresh (24 to 48 hour old) whole blood. If unavailable, then platelets, fresh frozen plasma, and cryoprecipitate are given slowly. Desmopressin acetate and epsilon aminocaproic acid (Amicar) are not routinely given unless coagulopathy is refractory to the measures described above. Antibiotics are given again after separation from CPB. Also, methylprednisolone (15 mg/kg) is given after protamine administration, and furosemide (1 mg/kg) is administered if urine output is < 1–2 cc/kg per hour. Patients are transported to the ICU with continuous monitoring of the ECG, arterial blood pressure, and oxygen saturation. Anesthesia is maintained in the ICU with continuous infusions of fentanyl (5 mcg/kg per hour) and vecuronium (0.1 mg/kg per hour) for the first 24 hours posttransplantation. The dose of fentanyl may be increased whenever there are signs of inadequate anesthesia since infants rapidly become tolerant to narcotic infusions.

Transplant Techniques for Hypoplastic Left Heart Syndrome (Type A)

Anesthesia is induced after the donor team confirms by visual inspection that the donor heart is acceptable. The recipient's skin incision should be timed to occur approximately 60 minutes before anticipated return of the donor heart. Through a median sternotomy incision, the pericardium is opened in the midline and reflected laterally. The head and neck vessels should be dissected and encircled with small vascular snares (Figure 12). Both pulmonary arteries are identified, dissected, and also encircled with vascular snares. The distal aorta beyond the arch vessels is also dissected

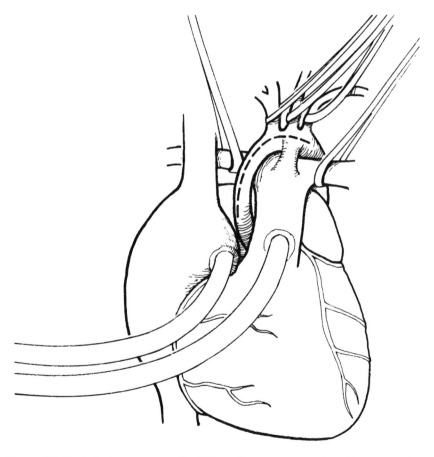

Figure 12. Recipient cannulation and line of aortic transection for Type A hypoplastic left heart syndrome.

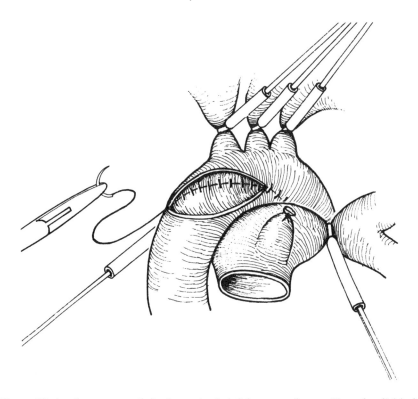

Figure 13. Aortic anastomosis for hypoplastic left heart syndrome. Note the divided ductus on the recipient pulmonary artery.

free and ensnared if possible. The ductus should be identified. Heparin is given and the right atrium is cannulated through the right atrial appendage (usually a 20 Fr catheter). The pulmonary artery is then cannulated (usually a 10 Fr arterial cannula).

When the donor heart has arrived in the operating room, CPB is established and the patient is cooled to 18°C. Both pulmonary arteries are ensnared as soon as CPB is begun. When the core body temperature reaches 18°C, circulatory arrest is begun, the head of the bed is lowered, and the head vessels are ensnared. The right atrial and pulmonary artery cannulae are removed.

The right atrium is divided in the usual fashion, with adequate tissue reserved for later right atrial anastomosis. The aorta is divided just above the aortic valve. The pulmonary artery and left atrium are divided as described for adult heart transplant. The lesser curvature of the recipient's aorta is opened along the undersurface of the arch. The ductus is divided and the pulmonary artery end is oversewn. The donor heart is prepared by excising the head and neck vessels from the donor aorta, and distally the donor aorta is divided at approximately the level of the ductal remnant. The anastomosis of the left atrium is then performed as for adult heart transplant (Figures 2 and 3), except that running 5–0 polypropylene suture is used. The right atrial anastomosis is performed next (Figure 4), also with running 5–0 polypropylene.

Next, the aortic anastomosis is performed to the undersurface of the recipient's aortic arch (Figure 13). The anastomosis is performed with running 6–0 polypropylene starting at the distal end of the anastomosis and suturing the back wall of the anastomosis first. The donor ascending aorta is

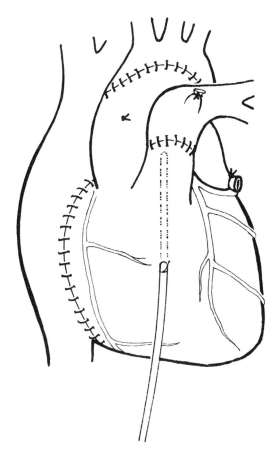

Figure 14. Completed transplant operation for hypoplastic left heart syndrome. A percutaneous catheter has been positioned in the main pulmonary artery.

then recannulated, and the donor right atrial appendage is cannulated. CPB is slowly restarted while the distal aorta snare is removed. Then the snares from the head vessels are removed. Flow is reestablished and the patient is rewarmed. The pulmonary artery anastomosis is performed with 6–0 polypropylene.

To manage pulmonary pressures postoperatively, we have found it helpful to place a percutaneous pulmonary artery pressure monitoring catheter through the proximal pulmonary artery. After the patient is rewarmed and effective cardiac contractions have resumed, CPB is weaned and the cannulas are removed after protamine is given (Figure 14). Because of the occasional marked size discrepancy with a much larger donor heart than the recipient's chest will accommodate, a temporary silastic patch may be used to close the skin incision without closing the underlying sternum. After myocardial edema has resolved, and hemodynamics have stabilized (usually 2–3 days), the chest can then be closed.

Appendix

Abbreviations

ICD = implantable cardioverter-defibrillator
Ao = aorta
AV = atrioventricular
CPB = cardiopulmonary bypass
CMV = cytomegalovirus
CVP = central venous pressure
DDAVP = desmopressin acetate
ECG = electrocardiogram
Fr = French
FRC = functional residual capacity
ICU = intensive care unit
IV = intravenous
IVC = inferior vena cava
NTG = nitroglycerine
PA = pulmonary artery
PFO = patent foramen ovale
PGE1 = prostaglandin E1
po = by mouth
PVR = pulmonary vascular resistance
SA = sinoatrial
SVC = superior vena cava

Selected References

1. Backer L, Idriss FS, Zales VR, et al. Cardiac transplantation for hypoplastic left heart syndrome: A modified technique. Ann Thorac Surg 1990;50:894–898.
2. Bailey LL. Heart transplantation techniques in complex congenital heart disease. J Heart Lung Transplant 1993;12:S168-S175.
3. Bailey LL, Gundry SR, Razzouk AJ, et al. Loma Linda University Pediatric Heart Transplant Group. Bless the babies: One hundred fifteen late survivors of heart transplantation during the first year of life. J Thorac Cardiovasc Surg 1993;105: 805–815.
4. Boucek MM, Mathis CM, Razzouk A, et al. Indications and contraindications for heart transplant in infancy. J Heart Lung Transplant 1993;12:S145-S148.
5. Burrows FA, Klinck JR, et al. Pulmonary hypertension in children: Perioperative management. Can Anaesth Soc J 1986;33:606–628.
6. Cannom DS, Rider AK, Stinson EB, et al. Electro-physiologic studies in the denervated transplanted human heart. II. Response to norepinephrine, isoproterenol and propranolol. Am J Cardiol 1975;36:859–866.
7. Carrel A, Guthrie CC. The transplantation of veins and organs. Am Med 1905;10:1101–1102.
8. Deleuze PH, Benvenuti C, Mazzucotelli JP, et al. Orthotopic cardiac transplantation with direct caval anastomosis: Is it the optimal procedure? J Thorac Cardiovasc Surg 1995;109:731–737.
9. Demas K, Wyner J, Mihm FG, et al. Anaesthesia for heart transplantation. A retrospective study and review. Br J Anaesth 1986;58:1357–1364.
10. Dreyfus G, Jebara VA, Couetil J, et al. Kinking of the pulmonary artery: A treatable cause of acute right ventricular failure after heart transplantation. J Heart Transplant 1990;9:575–576.
11. Dreyfus G, Jebara V, Mihailueanue S, et al. Total orthotopic heart transplantation: An alternative to the standard technique. Ann Thorac Surg 1991;52:1181–1184.
12. Emery JR. Strategies for prolonged survival before heart transplantation in the neonatal intensive care unit. J Heart Lung Transplant 1993;12:S161-S163.
13. Emery RW, Almquist AK, Von Rueden TJ, et al. Implantation of the implantable cardioverter defibrillator in the heart transplant candidate. J Heart Lung Transplant 1993;12:1067–1070.
14. Govier AV. Anesthesia and cardiac transplantation. In: Estafanous FG, ed. Anesthesia and the Heart Patient. Boston, Butterworths, 1989, pp. 99–107.
15. Grebenik CR, Robinon PN. Cardiac transplantation at Harefield. A review from the anaesthetist's standpoint. Anaesthesia 1985;40:131–140.
16. Hansen DD, Hickey PR. Anesthesia for hypoplastic left heart syndrome: Use of high-dose fentanyl in 30 neonates. Anesth Analg 1986;65:127–132.
17. Hickey PR, Hansen DD, Wessel GL, et al. Pulmonary and systemic hemodynamic responses to fentanyl in infants. Anesth Analg 1985;64:483–486.
18. Hickey PR, Hansen DD, Wessel GL, et al. Blunting of stress responses in the pulmonary circulation of infants by fentanyl. Anesth Analg 1985;64:1137.
19. Koehntop DE, Rodman JH, et al. Pharmacokinetics of fentanyl in neonates. Anesth Analg 1986;65:227–232.
20. Lewis AB, Freed MD, et al. Side effects of therapy with prostaglandin E1 in infants with critical congenital heart disease. Circulation 1981;64:893–898.

21. Lower RR, Stofer RC, Shumway NE. Homovital transplantation of the heart. J Thorac Cardiovasc Surg 1961;41:196–204.
22. Martin RD, Parisi F, et al. Anesthetic management of neonatal cardiac transplantation. J Cardiothorac Anesth 1989;3:465–469.
23. Mavroudis C, Harrison H, et al. Infant orthoptic cardiac transplantation. J Thorac Cardiovasc Surg 1988;96:912–924.
24. Mayer JE Jr. Cardiac transplantation for neonates with hypoplastic left heart syndrome. Ann Thorac Surg 1990;50:864–865.
25. Ream AK, Fowles RE, Jamieson S. Cardiac transplantation. In: Kaplan JA, ed. Cardiac Anesthesia. Second Edition. Philadelphia, WB Saunders, 1987, pp. 881–891.

Chapter 4

Routine Posttransplant Procedures and Early Postoperative Problems After Cardiac Transplantation

Patrick M. McCarthy, M.D., Edward B. Stinson, M.D.

The care of the cardiac transplant patient involves even more of a team effort than routine cardiac surgery. Although the transplant surgeon is responsible for the smooth working of all functions of the team, each member is also critically important. An experienced group of nurses, residents, physicians, and well-informed consultants is necessary to care for the multiple and complex problems that these patients may face.

Admission to the Intensive Care Unit

Room Cleaning and Isolation

Stanford is equipped with four laminar flow private rooms specifically designed for transplant patients, but these are generally reserved for heart-lung or lung transplant recipients. Heart transplant patients are usually placed in other intensive care unit (ICU) rooms, depending on the bed situation or nursing requirements. Patients are generally given a private room, although frequently transplant patients have stayed in the same room as other routine postoperative cardiac surgical patients (free of infection) without complications. Before the transplant patient is transferred from the operating room to the ICU, the furniture, equipment, and walls of the patient's room are thoroughly cleaned with Microbac or another antiseptic solution. Besides the usual cleaning, the ceiling vents are vacuumed, and the shades are washed.

Isolation procedures no longer require a mask, but thorough hand-washing is mandatory before personnel may enter the patient's room. More

From: Smith JA, McCarthy PM, Sarris GE, Stinson EB, Reitz BA (eds.): The Stanford Manual of Cardiopulmonary Transplantation. Futura Publishing Co., Inc., Armonk, NY, 1996.

63

extensive procedures are used if the patient's white blood count falls below 2,000/mm^3. No personnel or visitors with any known or suspected infectious disease are allowed into the room. The number of people who may enter the room is limited to reduce the amount of traffic in and out of the rooms. No fresh flowers are permitted in the room, and the doors and windows are kept closed. The patient is allowed to walk in the ICU or on the ward, but must wear a mask because of the risk of airborne infection.

Routine Orders

When the patient is transferred from the operating room, routine nursing orders are started. An electrocardiogram (ECG) and oxygen saturation monitors are placed. Vital signs, including central venous pressure (CVP), are measured every 20 minutes for 12 hours, then every 30 minutes for another 12 hours, then every 1 hour. Urine output and chest tube drainage are recorded every 30 minutes for 12 hours, and then every hour. An accurate intake and output are recorded every hour. CVP lines and pacing wires are cleaned and dressed daily. All intravenous (IV) tubing, bottles, and CVP manometers should be changed daily.

Initially, the CVP line and peripheral IV are maintained with fluids at a low rate to keep the lines open. The endotracheal tube is kept free of secretions with bagging and suctioning every 1 hour, and more often if needed. The patient should be turned every hour. The patients are maintained sedated initially and fully ventilated. As the patient awakens, if the transplanted heart and other organ systems are functioning well, then extubation may take place 12 hours after transplantation.

Initial routine lab work includes hematocrit, potassium, and blood gases every 4 hours. Daily lab tests include a complete blood count, platelet count, electrolytes, chemistry panel, prothrombin time, magnesium, and calcium. Cyclosporine levels are measured early every morning, and the results are usually available by noon. Twice a week a 12-hour urine creatinine clearance is performed. Once a week virology studies are done including cytomegalovirus (CMV) (IgG, IgM, and buffy coat viral culture) and urine and throat swabs for viral culture (shell vial assay). A portable chest film is taken immediately postoperatively and daily.

Postoperative Medications

Routine medications after transplantation include the usual postoperative medications following cardiac surgery. Morphine sulfate is given as needed for pain; occasionally midazolam is also required for sedation. Cefamandole (1 gm IV q 6 hours) is given for eight doses postoperatively. When the hemodynamic and volume status of the patient is stabilized, IV furosemide is given for diuresis. Usually the weight determined for an end-point is lower than the patient's preoperative weight because of preexisting congestive heart failure. It is usual for a patient to return to the ICU on a low dose of dopamine; frequently, nitroprusside is needed for hypertension and stable control of intravascular volume. Isoproterenol is often used to maintain the heart rate at 90–120 beats/minute during the first 48 hours to optimize cardiac output. Alternatively, atrial pacing may be used. Volume is given in the form of crystalloid or 5% albumin solution to maintain a CVP of 8–14 mmHg and mean arterial pressure > 60 mmHg. Blood is given to maintain a hematocrit > 30%.

Routine Problems After Transplantation

Postoperative Bleeding

As with all open heart operations, bleeding is sometimes a major concern. Before the patient leaves the operating room, a careful search for surgical bleeding sites is carried out. Even though a patient may have a known predisposition to abnormal bleeding, a surgical cause for the bleeding should always be kept in mind. Re-exploration for bleeding should not be delayed lest a surgical site be missed. In addition, heart transplant patients are at somewhat higher risk for postoperative coagulopathy. Most patients have taken warfarin before operation and its effects may not have been completely reversed by fresh frozen plasma given intraoperatively. Moreover, because of right heart failure, liver dysfunction may contribute to the postoperative bleeding.

Recently, we have routinely used prophylactic antifibrinolytic agents. Aprotinin (Trasylol) has most often been used in the context of a clinical investigation. Otherwise, high dose (30 gm) epsilon aminocaproic acid (Amicar) or high dose (10 gm) tranexamic acid (Cyclokapron) may be useful.

If the patient's prothrombin time is elevated after surgery, and oozing continues, then additional fresh frozen plasma and aquamephyton should be given. For patients on warfarin before surgery, aquamephyton is routinely given for the first 3 postoperative days.

Signs and symptoms of cardiac tamponade may be more difficult to interpret because of a denervated heart. The clinical clues of labile blood pressure, low urine output, and poor distal perfusion all suggest cardiac tamponade. A chest radiograph may show increased heart size, but tamponade may be present without this roentgenographic finding. Echocardiograms are of limited usefulness in determining this diagnosis. Because failure to treat cardiac tamponade and/or surgical bleeding may be disastrous, we recommend reoperation for a patient with these possible findings. The risks of reoperation are low.

Postoperative Changes

Patients may develop an active diuresis because of the high cardiac output of the transplanted heart, and they may need volume to stabilize the mean arterial pressure. A labile blood pressure may reflect autonomic dysfunction following cardiopulmonary bypass (CPB). Virtually all of these hemodynamic problems should respond to low doses of volume, inotropic drugs, or nitroprusside. For requirements beyond these, other causes should be sought.

Status II heart transplant patients have no unusual requirements for ventilation and respiration. They are typically extubated 12 hours after transplantation, depending upon their preoperative status, the type of anesthesia used, and the amount of postoperative sedation. Status I recipients in general are more debilitated and more overloaded with fluid before the operation and require longer periods of ventilator support after surgery. Managing arterial blood gases, pH, and blood chemistries are similar to the requirements of most postoperative heart cases. Hypokalemia should be aggressively treated, especially if diuresis is vigorous.

Special Problems After Transplantation: Hemodynamics

Right Heart Failure

Right heart failure is a common early problem following transplantation, and its etiology is usually multifactorial. Recipients with moderate elevations of pulmonary vascular resistance (PVR) are at high risk for this problem. Early in our experience, the mortality rate for patients with high PVR elevations was found to be excessive. The donor right ventricle (RV) may not be able to function effectively if the PVR is significantly elevated, especially if any hypoxemia or acidosis develops. This problem is sometimes seen also with donors who have sustained right ventricular myocardial contusions that were not readily apparent at organ retrieval.

The diagnosis of right heart failure is sometimes made at the transplant operation when the patient is being weaned from CPB. The RV may dilate, appear hypocontractile, and the CVP may rise. The pulmonary artery (PA) pressure is usually high. The PA pressure may be normal, or low, if the failing right heart is unable to generate a high pressure. More commonly today, because of better recipient and donor selection, right heart failure develops gradually over a period of hours in the ICU. It may be detected by elevated CVP, labile or low blood pressure, signs of poor peripheral perfusion, and new RV conduction delay.

If the diagnosis is made in the operating room, the PA anastomosis should be carefully inspected to ensure that no twisting or kinking of the anastomosis has occurred. Acute right ventricular failure that develops soon after weaning from bypass may be caused by an air embolus to the right coronary artery. This is usually transient and resolves with elevation of the perfusion pressure. In addition, a protamine reaction with pulmonary vasoconstriction may be considered in the differential diagnosis. Finally, an undetermined pulmonary embolus may have occurred since the recipient's initial evaluation. The PVR can be recalculated in the operating room using a PA catheter and left atrial (LA) pressure monitoring line. If the PVR is normal, a mechanical cause or RV contusion should be considered.

If the right heart failure is due to an elevated PVR, the situation may be improved by metabolic and pharmacologic manipulations (Table 1). The patient should be well oxygenated and not acidotic. Hyperventilation, to elevate the pH, should be started. Inotropic agents that tend to decrease the PVR, such as isoproterenol, dobutamine, and amrinone are frequently all that are needed.

For patients with more difficult problems and a fixed PVR, more po-

---

Table 1
Steps in the Management of Donor Right Heart Failure

1. Check PA anastomosis.
2. Consider coronary air embolus, pulmonary embolus, or protamine reaction.
3. Calculate PVR.
4. If PVR is normal, and no mechanical cause is found, start inotropic drugs.
5. If PVR is high:
   a. Hyperventilate (keep PH $\geq$ 7.5).
   b. Maintain pO_2 > 100 mmHg.
   c. Start (or increase) inotropic drugs/pulmonary vasodilators.
6. Administer prostaglandin E1.
7. Administer epinephrine and/or norepinephrine via LA line.
8. As "last resort" implant right ventricular assist device.

PA = pulmonary artery; PVR = pulmonary vascular resistance; LA = left atrial.

tent vasodilators are needed. In past years, we frequently used nitroglycerin as a vasodilator in this circumstance. However, recently we have been more successful using prostaglandin E_1 (PGE$_1$) as a pulmonary vasodilator, because the systemic effects of PGE$_1$ are less pronounced than those of nitroglycerin. PGE$_1$ is started with a usual dose of 25 ng/kg per min, then increased, as tolerated, up to doses of 100–200 ng/kg per min. In combination with epinephrine (e.g., 25 ng/kg per min), this pharmacologic treatment is usually satisfactory for most cases of donor right heart failure. Occasionally, an alpha-constrictor (norepinephrine) may be infused into the LA line, while PGE$_1$ is infused through the CVP line or a PA catheter.

In rare instances where the donor right heart failure will not respond to these treatments, mechanical support must be considered. In this circumstance, a right ventricular assist device may be used with venous inflow from the right atrium and return to the main PA. However, it is rare in these situations that this effort will be ultimately successful.

Biventricular Failure

Rarely, a patient will acutely develop biventricular failure after transplantation. This failure is ominous and usually indicates a more profound disorder than isolated right ventricular failure. It may be due to poor preservation of the graft or, more likely, to myocardial abnormalities present before graft harvesting (e.g., previous cardiac arrest, contusion, sepsis, and hypoxemia). Inotropic support with afterload reduction (pulmonary and systemic) is the mainstay of treatment, but intra-aortic balloon pumping may also be necessary. If all these measures fail to produce adequate cardiac output and graft function, biventricular assist devices should be placed. Although graft function may recover, the graft more likely will need to be promptly replaced, if the patient is to be salvaged. In that instance, the patient should be relisted (United Network for Organ Sharing [UNOS] Status I) for a second heart transplant.

Rarely, a condition that resembles biventricular failure in some respects may be caused by intraoperative sepsis attributable to active endocarditis (tricuspid valve or right atrium) in the donor graft. Usually *Staphylococcus aureus* is responsible, and vegetations will be identified when the donor right atrium is opened. These should be removed and stat gram stains obtained. The patient's resultant shock-like state is due to severe depression of systemic vascular tone. Treatment with appropriate antibiotics, volume, and inotropic and vasoconstrictor drugs will resolve the problem in most cases within 24–48 hours.

Hyperacute Rejection

Hyperacute rejection, one of the causes of acute biventricular failure, is very rare, but it should be considered in all cases. This catastrophic complication may be seen in a patient who has had a previous transplant or other surgery with preformed antibodies, or in a patient or who has received an ABO-incompatible graft due to clerical error. In these circumstances, the graft will show rapidly deteriorating function shortly after removal of the aortic cross-clamp. The graft becomes discolored and shows venous congestion. Pharmacologic efforts to support the patient are not adequate. Mechanical support should be used until another heart can be obtained for retransplantation.

Rhythm Disturbances

After heart transplantation, many patients initially have a junctional rhythm before sinus activity resumes. We prefer to maintain a heart rate of 90–120 beats/minute early after transplantation in order to optimize cardiac output. This can be done using either an isoproterenol drip or atrial pacing. A few patients (< 5%) will have permanent sinus node dysfunction. This condition is frequently associated with angiographically documentable injury to the sinus node artery, but other poorly understood factors also play a role. For these patients, a permanent pacemaker is usually implanted if the sinus node does not recover in 1 week. The type of pacemaker may be a VVI set at a backup rate so that it is used only during intermittent bradycardia. For most patients a rate-responsive pacemaker is implanted. We do not routinely use permanent atrial pacemakers in these patients (although others have) because of our concern about loss of atrial capture with time.

Occasionally, a patient develops supraventricular tachyarrhythmias as a result of mechanisms similar to those that follow routine open heart surgery. However, supraventricular tachyarrhythmias frequently indicate graft rejection. This possibility should be considered if the arrhythmia develops more than 5 days after transplantation. The late development of this rhythm is an indication for cardiac biopsy.

If pharmacologic treatment of atrial fibrillation or flutter is needed because of an excessively rapid ventricular response with impairment of cardiac output, verapamil is the drug of choice due to its prompt and direct action on the atrioventricular node. Digoxin may also be used in standard doses, but the rapid, vagally-mediated component of its effect will be absent. Only the direct depressant effect of digoxin on nodal conduction will be operative, and thus the lag time to full effect will be prolonged. Further, most recipients taking digoxin preoperatively will maintain measurable serum levels within or close to the "therapeutic range" for 2–4 days after operation, even though the drug was discontinued at the time of transplantation. Dosages, therefore, should be titrated accordingly.

Premature ventricular contractions, ventricular tachycardia, and ventricular fibrillation are very unusual following heart transplantation. If these occur early postoperatively, they are probably related to metabolic causes, such as hypokalemia, or to early graft failure with ventricular distention. Only in end-stage rejection do serious ventricular arrhythmias develop.

Early Postoperative Hypertension

Hypertension during the first several days after transplantation is common and the causes are multifactional. Typically, the transplanted heart provides a normal or elevated cardiac output, but the systemic vascular resistance remains elevated. Blood pressure control through neurogenic and hormonal mechanisms remains disturbed for days to weeks in most patients. In the first several days after transplantation, blood pressure control may be more of a problem in a small or moderate-sized patient who receives a relatively large graft. In pediatric transplant patients, this problem is even more common.

Initially, blood pressure is controlled with a nitroprusside drip. Gradually, over 2–3 days the problem usually resolves. The hypertension may contribute to headaches and nausea and vomiting. If nitroprusside is still required at 48 hours, then an oral antihypertensive agent is begun. Treatment is empiric at this point. Usually we would use an angiotensin-converting inhibitor and/or hydralazine and/or calcium channel blockers. Diltiazem is currently the drug of choice because of its protective effect regarding the development of graft coronary disease and also because it lowers the cyclosporine dosage requirement. Many patients who are hypertensive for the first few days gradually become normotensive, but approximately 75% of patients require antihypertensive therapy by 1 month.

Special Problems After Transplantation: Other Organ Systems

Renal Dysfunction

Urine output is typically copious in association with a newly increased cardiac output from the graft. Occasionally, however, preexisting renal disease, in combination with early cyclosporine administration and the dele-terious effects of CPB, will lead to marginal urine output. We no longer ad-minister cyclosporine preoperatively. When hemodynamics have stabilized and good urine output established, cyclosporine is started (usually on postop day 1 or 2) at low doses and titrated upwards gradually according to levels. Early oliguria is a serious problem because it may delay extubation, cause metabolic disorders, and progress to frank renal failure. Increasing doses of furosemide are indicated after it has been established that the in-travascular volume is adequate. Mannitol and bumetanide may be added if there is no response to furosemide. Nifedipine (10-mg sublingual) may be used, and sometimes dramatic improvement in urine output occurs be-cause the drug counteracts renal vasoconstriction induced by cyclosporine (other potentially effective drugs include misoprostol and pentoxifylline). If cyclosporine therapy was started prior to the development of oliguria, it should be stopped until resumption of normal, or near normal, renal func-tion. Withholding, reducing, or temporarily withdrawing cyclosporine at this early phase should not lead to acute rejection for patients who are re-ceiving prophylactic OKT3 (or other antilymphocyte preparations).

If acute renal failure develops, the usual supportive measures should be used (dialysis, medication adjustment, and reduced fluid intake). Cy-closporine is withheld, but, as it is not removed by dialysis, the levels grad-ually decline over a period of several days. Immunosuppression during this time is maintained with corticosteroids, azathioprine, and OKT3 during the first 14 days (see Chapter 6). As the patient nears the end of the 14-day course of OKT3, a low dose of cyclosporine may have to be reinstituted. In nearly all these early cases of acute renal failure, adequate renal function eventually resumes, albeit not at a totally normal level. It is very rare (< 1%) that permanent renal failure develops perioperatively (see Chapter 8).

Metabolic Abnormalities

Serum Calcium and Magnesium

As with any postoperative cardiac case, serum calcium should be mea-sured every 12 hours for the first 48 hours, and as needed after that. The ef-fects of cyclosporine on the kidneys may also lead to hypomagnesemia. Low magnesium levels can lead to arrhythmias, muscle cramps, irritability, and, occasionally, to seizures. Serum magnesium levels should be checked daily while the patient is in the hospital, and aggressive replacement given with IV magnesium sulfate or oral magnesium tablets.

Serum Glucose

Serum glucose should be checked every 8 hours for the first 48 hours after transplantation, and more often if indicated. After that, serum glucose should be checked daily. Hyperglycemia is common following transplantation, especially during the first 24 hours postoperatively when the patient has received large doses of steroids and catecholamine release is high. Additionally, patients are at risk during treatment of rejection episodes when they are given large increases of oral and IV steroids. In general, patients who are taking an oral antidiabetic agent before transplant surgery require insulin for several days or weeks after transplantation, and perhaps indefinitely thereafter. Many other patients will require insulin transiently, or perhaps the addition of an oral antidiabetic agent, during periods of high steroid usage.

Neurologic Complications

Headache

Headache is a very common complaint during the first several days after transplantation. It may be due to high cardiac output, hypertension, and/or narcotics for pain control. Frequently, it is associated with nausea and vomiting. Usually headache can be improved if not totally controlled by improvement of the blood pressure, gradual normalization of the cardiac output, and sedation. If the headaches are not responding to these measures, an infectious cause (see Chapter 7), or OKT3-induced aseptic meningitis should be considered. Some patients will require a head CT scan followed by a lumbar puncture. OKT3 meningitis, typically seen 3–5 days after the drug has been started, is associated with a sterile lymphocytosis of the cerebral spinal fluid. Viral cultures of the cerebrospinal fluid should be evaluated to differentiate viral meningitis from OKT3 meningitis.

Seizures

Some patients will develop seizures, which are frequently associated with severe headaches. These seizures may be caused by high cardiac output with cerebral hyperperfusion, or by other medications or metabolic causes. The usual metabolic causes should be sought (serum glucose, electrolytes, calcium, and phosphorus), and hypomagnesemia should be excluded. These patients require an emergency head CT scan, neurology consultation, and frequently, lumbar puncture. If seizures occur very early after transplantation, they may be related to the operation and either atheroma or air may have caused cerebral emboli. In most patients with seizures, however, no specific cause can be identified. Although anti-epileptic agents may be withheld if an isolated seizure occurs very early postoperatively, more delayed occurrence of seizures, or recurrent seizures, should prompt therapy with phenytoin (dilantin).

Mental Status

The mental status of most posttransplant patients is normal for a postoperative cardiac patient. Some patients will be somnolent, perhaps because of preexisting liver dysfunction and an inability to clear analgesics. Psychological problems are very common, despite extensive preoperative screening. Patients have been experiencing a sustained period of stress while awaiting transplant surgery, and decompensation after the operation is not unusual. It is exacerbated by steroid use and may be made especially worse after bolus treatments for rejection. An appropriate psychiatric consultation should be obtained. However, the choice of antipsychotic medication, if any, should be carefully reviewed because of the associated cardiac effects of some of these drugs.

Tremor

Many patients will notice a fine, sometimes even coarse, tremor, which is a side effect of cyclosporine treatment. The tremor is worse when higher doses of cyclosporine are given in the early posttransplant period, but in most patients it gradually resolves. In and of itself a tremor does not require extensive workup, but patients should be reassured that it is a medication side effect that should improve with time.

Gastroenterologic Problems

Nausea and Vomiting

Nausea and vomiting are frequently seen in the early posttransplantation period. These may be related to narcotics or to the immunosuppressants (especially cyclosporine or OKT3). In most patients, the symptoms are self-limited and resolve gradually over 2–3 days. Antiemetics may be useful for symptomatic relief. Should symptoms persist or be associated with abdominal pain, peptic ulcer disease, pancreatitis, or bowel obstruction should be considered.

Diarrhea

Diarrhea may also occur in the early postoperative period. Pseudomembranous enterocolitis should be excluded by performing stool cultures and having a stool specimen tested for *Clostridium difficile* titers. Stool cultures for other pathogens (e.g., *Salmonella, Shigella*) should also be tested, as well as stool cultures for ova and parasites. Neutropenic colitis should also be considered in the differential diagnosis in a patient who has a correspondingly low white blood cell count. Colitis secondary to CMV infection also has been seen. These diagnoses are best confirmed by colonoscopy with tissue biopsy.

Peptic Ulcers

Peptic ulcer disease may develop because of the concomitant steroid use and high stress of the perioperative period. We use antacids for ulcer prophylaxis (30 cc tid). For patients who are at particularly high risk ranitidine may be used, in preference to cimetidine, because of less interference with cyclosporine metabolism. Intra-abdominal emergencies requiring operative treatment are most often related to complications of peptic ulcer disease, diverticulitis, or other bowel perforation. In the event of such an intra-abdominal catastrophe, we prefer to minimize steroids, decrease azathioprine, and maintain immunosuppression primarily with cyclosporine.

Pancreatitis

Pancreatitis may be related to the use of steroids or cyclosporine. In addition, it is sometimes seen after routine cardiac surgery. We perform serum amylase determinations twice a week for the first 2 weeks, even though the patients may not have symptoms. The early detection of pancreatitis may help to avoid more significant problems. If pancreatitis develops, the patient should be kept NPO (nothing by mouth) and a CT scan performed to document the extent of the problem. The management of pancreatitis is similar to that given to nontransplant patients, i.e., medical therapy primarily, and withholding of surgical intervention unless complications develop.

Liver Dysfunction

Liver dysfunction may develop early after transplantation and is usually multifactorial. Many patients have preexisting severe right heart failure and mild hepatic insufficiency. Azathioprine and cyclosporine can both lead to further liver dysfunction. Liver function tests are obtained at least 2–3 times a week during the initial month after transplantation. Should liver dysfunction develop, cyclosporine doses should be adjusted downward and azathioprine may need to be reduced. Alternative causes for liver dysfunction (e.g., gallstones, other drug reaction, and viral hepatitis, including CMV) should be excluded.

Miscellaneous Complications After Transplantation

Pleural Effusions

Pleural effusions are common before transplant surgery due to congestive heart failure. They should be drained at the time of transplantation. However, some patients will develop effusions after surgery. These should be removed by thoracentesis or chest tube if necessary. Effusions should be submitted for appropriate biochemical analysis and broad spectrum cultures. Occasionally, pleural effusions after transplantation are associated with otherwise unrecognized pulmonary emboli. These are seen more commonly in patients who are hospitalized and very debilitated before transplantation.

Pericardial Effusions

Pericardial effusions are frequently encountered after transplant surgery. They may be typical serosanguineous effusions such as are found after routine open heart operations, or they may result from accumulation of lymphatic fluid due to the extensive dissection near the aorta and pulmonary arteries. Pericardial effusions can be identified by increased heart size on postoperative chest radiographs and confirmed by echocardiography. If the effusion is very large or associated with any evidence of impaired cardiac filling, it should be evacuated. Pericardiocentesis may be acceptable therapy, but surgical drainage may be required for more recalcitrant effusions. A few patients have required late reoperation because they developed pericardial effusions, often in association with acute graft rejection. In these cases, we create a large pericardial window (via left anterolateral thoracotomy) with drainage into the pleural space. The finding of a pericardial friction rub on physical examination soon after transplant surgery is common, but it is always evanescent unless acute rejection intervenes.

Respiratory Function

Because patients with significant lung disease are excluded from selection for cardiac transplantation, the respiratory status of transplant patients is usually as good as, or better than, that of general cardiac surgery patients. Nevertheless, because of their debilitated state, all transplant patients are started on aggressive respiratory therapy, including incentive spirometers and chest physiotherapy, for 48 hours after extubation. Patients are also encouraged to walk frequently as soon as possible. Respiratory failure is rarely due to isolated pulmonary causes but, more commonly, to combination of other posttransplant complications, such as neurologic dysfunction or sepsis.

Physical Conditioning

Starting early after transplantation, patients are encouraged to increase their range and level of activities. Even young patients may have been very inactive during the wait before transplantation. Progressive physical reconditioning should be instituted with the help of the physical therapy department. Patients are encouraged to walk and ride stationary bicycles. By the time they leave the hospital, patients are able to comply with this regimen and continue their conditioning after discharge.

Other complications related to the immunosuppressive medications, rejection, and infection are discussed in Chapters 6, 7, and 8.

Routine Posttransplant Recovery

The routine posttransplant patient is hospitalized for 8–10 days (Table 2). The early ICU stay is spent recuperating from the operation. During the

Table 2
Routine Posttransplant Recovery: The First 14 Days

Postoperative Day	Activity
0	Operation; to ICU.
1	Extubated; up in bed.
2	Chest tubes removed; up in room; start physical therapy.
3	Wean drips.
4	Ambulate in ICU; learn medication instructions.
5–7	Out of ICU to intermediate care. Physical therapy and education begin. Discharge planning.
7	Biopsy.
8–10	Continued physical therapy and education. If biopsy negative, discharge to Home-Tel.
11–20	Outpatient management, follow-up in transplant clinic.
13	Biopsy and predischarge arteriogram.
14	Complete OKT3; home if biopsy negative.

next phase, when the patient is transferred to intermediate care, the patient and family are trained by the nursing staff about transplant medication schedules and side effects. The patient undergoes one cardiac biopsy, on postoperative day 7, and, if no rejection is found, the patient is discharged from the hospital. Patients remain close to the hospital for a few days after discharge, frequently at an apartment complex (the "Home-Tel") adjacent to the hospital. They receive the remainder of the 14-day course of OKT3 (and 4- to 6-week course of gancyclovir) as outpatients. The 2-week routine biopsy and baseline coronary arteriogram are obtained just prior to discharge, if convalescence has been slower, but are otherwise performed on an outpatient basis. The arteriogram provides a baseline for comparison with subsequent yearly studies to evaluate the transplanted heart for the development of coronary artery disease.

Selected References

1. Armitage J, Hardesty RL, Griffith BP. Prostaglandin E1: An effective treatment of right heart failure after orthotopic heart transplantation. J Heart Transplant 1987;6:348–351.
2. Banner NR, Yacoub MH. Physiology of the orthotopic cardiac transplant recipient. Semin Thorac Cardiovasc Surg 1990;2:259–270.
3. D'Ambra MN, LaRaia PJ, Philbin DM, et al. Prostaglandin E1: A new therapy for refractory right heart failure and pulmonary hypertension after mitral valve replacement. J Thorac Cardiovasc Surg 1985;89:567–572.

4. DiSesa VJ, Kirkman RL, Tilney NL. Management of general surgical complications following cardiac transplantation. Arch Surg 1989;124:539–541.
5. Dresdale A, Diehl J. Early postoperative care: Infectious disease considerations. Prog Cardiovasc Dis 1990;33(1):1–9.
6. Farrell TG, Camm AJ. Action of drugs in the denervated heart. Semin Thorac Cardiovasc Surg 1990;2:279–289.
7. Heerdt PM, Weiss CI. Prostaglandin E1 and intrapulmonary shunt in cardiac surgical patients with pulmonary hypertension. Ann Thorac Surg 1990;49:463–465.
8. Heinz G, Hirschl MM, Kratochwill C, et al. Inducibe atrial flutter and fibrillation after orthotopic heart transplantation. J Heart Lung Transplant 1993;12:517–521.
9. Hess W, Arnold B, Veit S. The haemodynamic effects of amrinone in patients with mitral stenosis and pulmonary hypertension. Eur Heart J 1986;7:800.
10. Hines RL. Management of acute right ventricular failure. J Card Surg 1990;5(Suppl 1):285–287.
11. Iberer F, Wasler A, Tscheliessnigg K, et al. Prostaglandin E_1-induced moderation of elevated pulmonary vascular resistance. Survival on waiting list and results of orthotopic heart transplantation. J Heart Lung Transplant 1993;12:173–178.
12. Kieler-Jenson N, Milocco I, Ricksten S-E. Pulmonary vasodilation after heart transplantation: A comparison among prostacyclin, sodium nitroprusside, and nitroglycerin on right ventricular function and pulmonary selectivity. J Heart Transplant 1993;12:179–184.
13. Kirklin JK, Naftel DC, Kirklin JW, et al. Pulmonary vascular resistance and the risk of heart transplantation. J Heart Transplant 1988;7:331–336.
14. Liem BL, DiBiase A, Schroeder JS. Arrhythmias and clinical electrophysiology of the transplanted human heart. Semin Thorac Cardiovasc Surg 1990;2:271–278.
15. Martin MA, Massanari RM, Nghiem DD, et al. Nosocomial aseptic meningitis associated with administration of OKT3. JAMA 1988;259:2002–2005.
16. Morley D, Boigon M, Fesniak H, et al. Posttransplantation hemodynamics and exercise function are not affected by body-size matching of donor and recipient. J Heart Lung Transplant 1993;12:770–778.
17. Odom NJ, Richens D, Glenville BE, et al. Successful use of mechanical assist device for right ventricular failure after orthotopic heart transplantation. J Heart Transplant 1990;9:652–653.
18. Redmond JM, Zeher KJ, Gillinov MA, et al. Use of theophylline for treatment of prolonged sinus node dysfunction in human orthotopic heart transplantation. J Heart Lung Transplant 1993;12:133–139.
19. Steck TB, Durkin MG, Costanzo-Nordin MR, et al. Gastrointestinal complications and endoscopic findings in transplant patients. J Heart Lung Transplant 1993;12:244–251.
20. Walsh TR, Guttendorf J, Dummer S, et al. The value of protective isolation procedures in cardiac allograft recipients. Ann Thorac Surg 1989;47:493–498.

Chapter 5

Mechanical Circulatory Support in the Bridge-to-Transplant Patient

Patrick M. McCarthy, M.D.,
Julian A. Smith, M.B., M.S., FRACS,
Philip E. Oyer, M.D., Ph.D., Peer M. Portner, Ph.D.

A patient accepted for cardiac transplantation must sometimes wait a long time before a donor becomes available. During this wait, a patient may die suddenly. Of those who have died waiting for transplants at Stanford University, almost half were sudden deaths. Antiarrhythmic drugs and the selective use of the implantable cardioverter defibrillator may decrease the risk of sudden death during this waiting period.

Other patients experience a decline in ventricular function and functional status during this period. These patients can be hospitalized, started on intravenous inotropic drugs, and reclassified as Status I (United Network for Organ Sharing [UNOS] criteria) to expedite their transplantation status. Some Status I patients, however, continue to deteriorate and require mechanical circulatory support to avoid compromising other organ systems or to prevent death. Another group of patients are sometimes referred late in their clinical course or experience acute decompensation (after myocardial infarction), and require emergency inotropic, and sometimes mechanical support, during their evaluation for heart transplant.

Several pumps have been designed to support the circulation, but they vary in their degree of invasiveness, complexity, and effectiveness. This chapter outlines our strategy for evaluating patients as candidates for circulatory support, our decisions regarding the type of pump to be used, our management of these patients, and our results with circulatory support in the bridge-to-transplant period.

From: Smith JA, McCarthy PM, Sarris GE, Stinson EB, Reitz BA (eds.): The Stanford Manual of Cardiopulmonary Transplantation. Futura Publishing Co., Inc., Armonk, NY, 1996.

Evaluation of Candidates for Bridge-to-Transplant

Indications for Circulatory Support

The proper time to initiate mechanical support is often difficult to define. Delaying until the patient is moribund yields poor results. On the other hand, intervening with expensive, invasive devices knowing that a donor heart could become available at any time is difficult. In general, erring on the side of early implantation is advisable because after a certain level of decompensation the patient may not be able to recover in time.

Once the patient is Status I, pharmacologic support is used as needed. Our patients are typically supported with dopamine and/or dobutamine. An afterload reducer (nitroprusside) is frequently helpful, and we use epinephrine only if more inotropic effect is needed. Amrinone offers some theoretic benefits, but its usefulness is limited by the thrombocytopenia that accompanies chronic administration. Milrinone may be preferable as the risk of thrombocytopenia is significantly less.

Table 1 lists our criteria for determining if mechanical support should be added to the maximal drug therapy. These patients have a low cardiac index and elevated left atrial (LA) pressure typical of end-stage heart failure. Many have symptomatic pulmonary edema and may need intubation and mechanical ventilation. The patient may have decreased mental activity and be very somnolent. Urine output may be falling and creatinine rising. Later, metabolic acidosis and ventricular arrhythmias occur and require prompt mechanical support because of the high risk of sudden death.

Table 1
Indications and Contraindications for Circulatory Support

Indications	Contraindications
Acceptable for heart transplant*	Unacceptable for heart transplant*
Receiving maximal pharmacologic support	Sepsis
Cardiac index < 2.0 L/min per m_2	Coma
Left atrial pressure > 20 mmHg	Anuria
Metabolic acidosis	Multiorgan failure syndrome
Decreased mental status	
Pulmonary edema	
Rising creatinine values	
Life-threatening arrhythmias	

*See Chapter 1.

Other considerations in timing the initiation of mechanical support are related to nonhemodynamic factors. These include the patients blood group, height, and weight, pulmonary vascular resistance, previous cardiac operations, position on the UNOS list, and "typical" local donor availability. A large blood type O recipient with elevated pulmonary vascular resistace can expect a long wait before a donor becomes available, even as Status I.

Is the Patient (Still) a Candidate for Transplantation?

Patients are sometimes referred in critical condition, especially after acute myocardial infarction, and a rapid evaluation is needed to determine the overall suitability for transplantation (see the criteria described in Chapter 1). Patients already accepted for transplantation must be reevaluated because contraindications may have developed (Table 1). For these critically ill patients, sepsis is a major concern and should be investigated before bridging is attempted. Typically, because patients are in the intensive care unit (ICU) and immobile, they are at high risk for pulmonary and line sepsis. All attempts should be made to clear infections in a Status I patient as soon as possible because sepsis is a strong contraindication to transplantation and mechanical circulatory support.

The most difficult clinical question frequently centers around the "reversibility" of other organ system function. Although we have successfully bridged patients with decreased mental status, we would not bridge a patient in frank coma because of the low likelihood for success. We attempt to intervene when renal function starts to deteriorate; however, if anuria has supervened, the chances of renal function returning are diminished. The patient may also have other organ dysfunction, such as hepatic dysfunction, coagulopathy, or metabolic disturbances. Usually, a patient will not be excluded from consideration for circulatory support based on one criterion only. The chances for success are low with multiorgan failure syndrome, and moribund patients are poor candidates for bridging. Nevertheless, it is always difficult to determine when a patient has become irreversibly moribund.

Intra-Aortic Balloon Pump

Many patients can be stabilized just by the insertion of an intra-aortic balloon pump (IABP) (Table 2). For acutely decompensated patients who

Table 2
Comparison of Circulatory Support Pumps for
Bridge-to-Transplant Patients

Criteria	Intra-aortic Balloon Pump	Centrifugal Pump	Novacor Pump
Advantages	Readily available Relatively inexpensive Easily placed and removed Does not preclude LVAD	Uni- and biventricular support Suitable for smaller patients Easily placed after cardiotomy Preferred to pulsatile pumps	Very effective Patient is mobile Wearable (totally implantable?) Flexible programming
Disadvantages	Less effective than LVAD Ineffective for severe RV failure Contraindicated for aortic insufficiency Immobilizes patient Risk of leg ischaemia	Invasive Flow generally less than with pulsatile pumps Low dose anticoagulation Possible embolization Pump head changes Limited patient mobility	Cost Size Noise Anticoagulation Very invasive Still experimental

LVAD = left ventricular assist device; RV = right ventricular.

have not been fully evaluated as transplant candidates, the IABP may allow more time to assess their condition. Balloon pumps are readily available in most centers and usually are easily placed and removed. If the patient is judged not to be a transplant candidate, then the IABP can be removed with little difficulty, in contrast to a ventricular assist device.

The IABP has several disadvantages. First, it is not as effective as more sophisticated circulatory support devices, especially for patients with severe right heart failure. It should not be used in a patient with aortic insufficiency. If it has been placed through the femoral artery, the patient cannot be mobilized and ambulate while awaiting transplant; as a result, the patient is more prone to respiratory infections, deep venous thrombosis, and other problems that may preclude transplant. Finally, leg ischemia is a significant risk in patients with borderline cardiac output. At Stanford we insert an IABP if the patient has had borderline decompensation with inotropic drugs, and we do not anticipate a long wait before a donor organ becomes available.

Centrifugal Pumps for Ventricular Assistance

Pump Design and Function

One advantage of the centrifugal pump over other ventricular assist systems is its functional simplicity. Located outside the patient, the pump contains a series of impellers that are turned by electromagnetic force supplied by the console. The rate of flow depends on the revolutions per minute imparted to the pump head, the preload, and resistance to outflow (afterload). Blood is routed through a cannula from the heart chambers to the apex of the pump head (inflow) and is pumped from the side of the pump head through a second cannula to the ascending aorta (outflow). Centrifugal pumps are commercially available and are not considered experimental, although they are not FDA approved for use as a bridge-to-transplant.

Indications for Use

Patients considered for mechanical support using a centrifugal pump as a bridge-to-transplant meet the guidelines outlined in Table 1. The centrifugal pump is useful for smaller adults and children; for larger adult patients we prefer to use an implantable assist system, such as the Novacor Left Ventricular Assist System (Baxter Healthcare, Novacor Division, Oakland, CA, USA), whenever possible. The greatest experience with centrifugal pumps is in their use in post-cardiotomy patients who cannot be successfully weaned from cardiopulmonary bypass. Insertion, maintenance, and complications of the device are the same in post-cardiotomy and bridge-to-transplant patients. However, for post-cardiotomy patients, the goal is to remove the pump when the heart has recovered, whereas for the bridge-to-transplant patient, the goal is to support the patient until a transplant is possible. Occasionally, post-cardiotomy patients who cannot be weaned from the pump are accepted for transplant, and the pump functions as a bridge-to-transplant. Similarly, the device has been placed in patients who have sustained a massive myocardial infarction. If cardiac function improves after recovery on the pump, it is removed; otherwise, the pump can be used as a bridge if the patient is accepted as a transplant candidate.

Univentricular and Biventricular Support

Whether to use a left ventricular assist device (LVAD) or a biventricular assist (BiVAD) is sometimes a difficult decision. Heart transplant candidates have been selected because their pulmonary artery pressures and pulmonary vascular resistance are near normal or only moderately elevated at pretransplant testing. Usually, only left ventricular (LV) support is sufficient because blood can flow through the lungs, even with severe right ventricular (RV) dysfunction.

Some patients (approximately 20%) may require additional support for the right ventricle (RVAD) because of transient increases in pulmonary vascular resistance. The etiology and treatment of right heart failure after LVAD insertion is similar to that seen after heart transplantation, as outlined in Chapter 4 (see Table 1 of Chapter 4). Increased pulmonary vascular resistance typically has several causes. Before LVAD insertion, it may be caused by pulmonary edema, acidosis, and/or hypoxemia. At the time of LVAD insertion, it may transiently worsen due to the effects of cardiopulmonary bypass and the administration of perioperative fluid, blood, and blood products. These patients may require biventricular support until the damage to the lungs improves. Then the RVAD can be weaned and removed, usually within a few days.

Isolated RV mechanical support is rarely used in the bridge-to-transplant patient, even in post-cardiotomy patients. In general, patients who require isolated RV support have a pulmonary vascular resistance above the acceptable level for orthotopic heart transplant.

Inserting Cannulas for the Centrifugal Pump

Cannulas for the pump are inserted through a median sternotomy incision while the patient is on cardiopulmonary bypass. For blood inflow to the pump we prefer a large (usually 32 Fr) cannula with a "lighthouse" tip or one of the right angle cannulas designed specifically for circulatory support (DLP Products, Grand Rapids, MI, USA). Their tips are less likely to occlude against the atrial (or ventricular) wall. The LA cannula is usually placed through a small incision in the right superior pulmonary vein within the pericardium. The tip of the cannula can be positioned in the posterior left atrium or across the mitral valve into the left ventricle. For outflow back to the patient, a 9 mm Gott shunt (Argyle Co., St. Louis, MO, USA) or any other standard arterial cannula used for cardiopulmonary bypass can be used. We prefer the Gott shunt because its length can easily be adjusted by cutting the cannula and it is long enough to connect to the pump line outside the chest. Cannulating the ascending aorta (rather than femoral artery) for outflow reduces the risk of leg ischemia. Similar cannulas for RVAD support are placed into the right atrium, and either the main pulmonary artery or RV outflow tract.

The cannulas are placed through stab wounds in the lower chest so that the sternum and incision can be closed (Figure 1). Chest closure decreases the risk of mediastinitis and also is important for extubating the patient. The lines and the pump head can be filled with saline in a large basin and then connected to the cannulas, or, preferably, they can be filled by

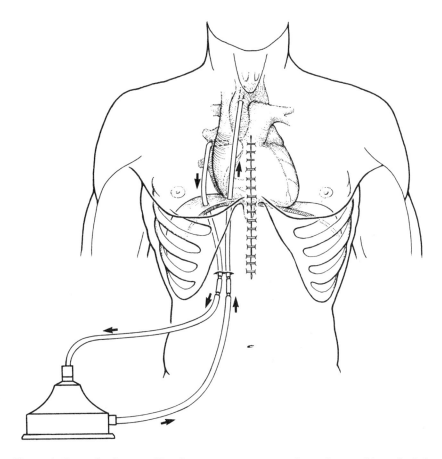

Figure 1. Cannulas for centrifugal pumps most commonly are inserted into the left atrium via the right superior pulmonary vein and into the ascending aorta. If possible the chest incision is closed. The pump head is outside the patient's body.

back-bleeding once the arterial cannula is placed and connected. Either way it is critically important to search carefully for air bubbles (especially where they become trapped in the pump head) before the pump begins to operate. Once the cannulas are inserted, purse-string sutures are tied around the insertion sites and secured around the cannulas. The cannulas are also carefully secured to the patient externally to avoid accidental dislodgment. The lines must be clamped until the pump is ready to start; otherwise, blood will flow retrograde from the high pressure systemic circulation to the left atrium!

A small atrial septal defect, or patent foramen ovale (PFO), may lead to life-threatening hypoxemia for a patient on LVAD support. Right-to-left shunt at the atrium level should be considered for any LVAD patient with hypoxemia. Some surgeons routinely inspect the atrial septum before pump insertion to avoid this problem. Intraoperative transesophageal echocardiography can also be used to diagnose the PFO before LVAD insertion.

While the LVAD is functioning, negative pressure may develop in the left atrium during periods of high flow. Air may be sucked into the left atrium around the cannula insertion site. The air will enter the pump head (Figure 2) and can be heard or felt as "chatter" as it embolizes. This prob-

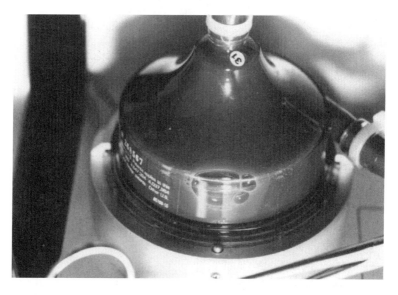

Figure 2. Large air pockets were seen in the pump head of the centrifugal LVAD. The patient became hypovolemic, and "chatter" was felt in the pump head before it was changed.

lem should be avoided during the operation, and is most often seen while "drying up."

If a BiVAD is used, flow is first established in the LVAD, and the RVAD is then gradually started and the flow is adjusted in both. As flow is established, cardiopulmonary bypass is gradually discontinued. Protamine is given when adequate flow (≥ 3.0 L/min) is established.

Achieving hemostasis can be a major problem, especially in postcardiotomy patients, but it is mandatory for success. Surgical bleeding must be stopped, hypothermia has to be corrected, coagulopathy must be rapidly treated with blood products, and pharmacologic agents must be used to decrease bleeding (e.g., aminocaproic acid or aprotinin). Transfusion of multiple units of blood and blood products may lead to pulmonary dysfunction and subsequent right heart failure. While LV support may have been required initially, RV support may have to be added later. Pulmonary vasodilators and inotropic drugs are usually given routinely perioperatively for RV support to help avoid this problem (see Chapter 4).

Adjusting Flow with the Centrifugal Pump

One major advantage of the centrifugal pump over more complicated implantable assist devices is its simplicity of operation. If the cannulas have been placed properly so that they drain well (without kinking or occluding against the wall of the atrium), then flow is generally easy to adjust. The speed (revolutions per minute [rpm]) of the impellers can be increased or lowered to adjust the flow, as measured by an in-line sensor. We try to obtain a cardiac index $\geq 2.0 - 2.5$ L/min per m². In general, this value can be obtained with 3,000 rpms. When the rpms are too high, flow no longer increases but starts to fluctuate as the lines begin to "chatter" or shake. The rpms should be maintained at the lowest acceptable level to minimize blood trauma and avoid the creation of air via cavitation (such as the bubbles around the propellers of a submarine).

The centrifugal pump system is nonocclusive. Therefore, if flow is stopped (e.g., to run a cardiac output or remove the pump), one of the lines *must be clamped*. Otherwise, blood will flow from the high pressure chamber (i.e., aorta) to the low pressure chamber (i.e., left atrium) with disastrous consequences. The lines may be clamped while the pump head is turning (unlike a roller pump) without risk of line separation.

When adequate flow cannot be obtained at the expected rpms, the problem is usually hypovolemia, which is manifested by line chatter and variation in the flow rate at a previously steady rpm. The flow usually stabilizes but at a lower level when the rpms are reduced. If central venous pressure (CVP) is low (or lower than previously), then volume loading usually corrects the pressure and flow increases. If the CVP is rising, then pulmonary vascular resistance may have risen with secondary RV failure. Monitoring both CVP and direct LA measurements (via a percutaneous LA line) simplifies the diagnosis and management of postoperataive hemodynamics. If both CVP and LA pressures are low, the problem is hypovolemia and should respond to volume replacement. If the CVP is high and LA pressure low then right heart failure is likely, and should be treated with pulmonary vasodilators, etc. as discussed in Chapter 4. If both CVP and LA are high and flow is down, the problem may be cardiac tamponade, or overexpansion of the noncompliant edematous lungs. This may respond to ventilator changes to decrease tidal volume and increase respiratory rate. Cardiac tamponade must be treated by prompt reoperation.

Anticoagulation

Patients on centrifugal pump support are at risk of clot formation with embolization from the pump head, the cannulas, and poorly contracting cardiac chambers (especially the left ventricle). Using protamine to reverse heparin is almost always necessary to obtain hemostasis. As soon as bleeding subsides, however, an infusion of low dose heparin should be started (to maintain an activated clotting time of 150–200 seconds) and continued while the pump is in place. In addition, low flow should be avoided.

Pump Head Replacement

After several days, the pump head may develop a vibration that can indicate impending failure. If this vibration develops, the head should be replaced immediately. Some programs routinely replace the pump head every 5–7 days during prolonged support to avoid problems. Two spare heads should always be kept near the pump when it is in use.

The pump head can be changed in < 2 minutes if the team is experienced and prepared. A small bolus of heparin is usually given first and resuscitation drugs should be kept nearby. The inflow and outflow lines are clamped as the pump is turned off. The pump head is removed from the console, and the lines are prepped with betadine and cut with sterile heavy scissors near their connections to the head. The pump outflow (arterial) line is connected first, and the new pump head is filled by back-bleeding. An air-free connection is then made to the pump inflow (LA) line. The new pump head is replaced in the console and the clamps removed as flow is reestablished.

Pump Explant and Heart Transplantation

In contrast to implantable assist devices, removing the cannulas of the centrifugal pump for heart transplantation is straight forward. Care must be taken to avoid dislodgment and air entry into the lines during prepping and opening. The patient is cannulated for cardiopulmonary bypass in the standard fashion for transplantation. The cannulas are removed after cardiopulmonary bypass has started, and the remainder of the operation is routine.

Implantable Left Ventricular Mechanical Support: The Novacor Pump

Pump Design and Function

The Novacor pump is still experimental and available at only a few medical centers. Because of its limited availability, the details of its set-up and operation are not included in this chapter.

The electrically powered Novacor pump is implanted in the abdominal wall and is capable of LV circulatory support. A pusher plate mechanism is used to pump the blood, and the inflow and outflow valves are made from bovine pericardium. Inflow into the pump comes from the LV apex, and outflow to the patient is through a graft into the aorta. The pump is connected to the drive console by a cable that passes through a percutaneous vent. A 20-foot cable connects the pump to the drive console and allows the patient to be mobile while connected to the pump (Figure 3). A new "wearable" Novacor is now available with portable external battery power (Figure 4). The wearable Novacor system affords the patient greater mobility and quality of life.

When operating normally, the pump is filled to a maximum stroke volume of 73 mL (Figure 3). Pump ejection is triggered when the rate of pump fill falls below an adjustable threshold near the end of native LV systole. Once set, the system is self-adjusting over a wide range of heart rates and stroke volumes. During normal operation, the LV pressure is usually substantially lower than the systemic pressure; consequently, the native aortic valve rarely opens while the pump is operating.

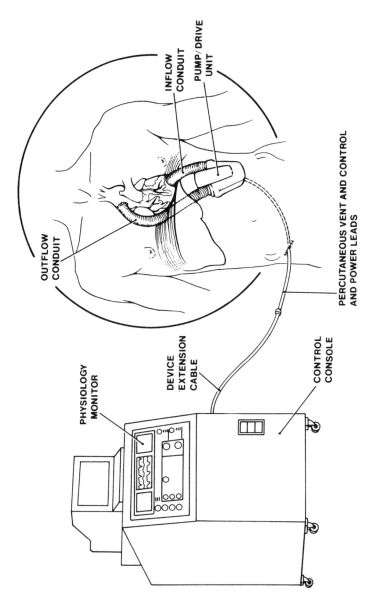

Figure 3. The Novacor pump is attached by a 20-foot drive cable to the portable control console. Reproduced with permission from McCarthy PM, et al. Clinical experience with the Novacor ventricular assist system: Bridge-to-transplant and the transition to chronic application. J Thorac Cardiovasc Surg 1991;102:578–587.

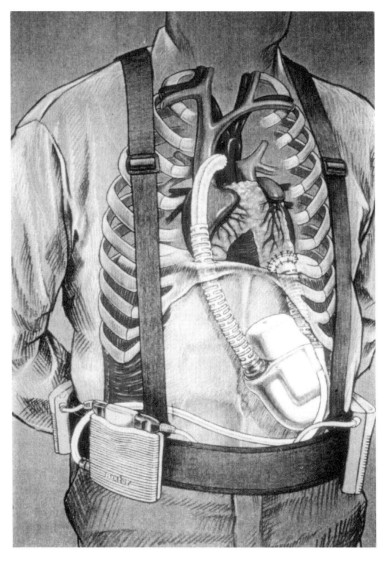

Figure 4. The "wearable" Novacor pump with the compact controller and batteries worn on a belt.

Patient Selection

Candidates for the Novacor pump include all patients who require mechanical circulatory assistance, as outlined in Table 1. Typically these are Status I patients waiting for heart transplants who progressively deteriorate on inotropic drugs. Although most patients deteriorate, they do not need to have an IABP implanted first, as it limits mobility and is a less attractive long-term option for most patients.

The major limitation of using the Novacor pump is usually the size of the patient. An abdominal wall of an adequate size to easily accommodate the pump requires that most patients must have a body surface area of at least 1.5 m². The majority of such patients are adult men, although we are able to implant the pump in a postpartum woman because of her slack abdominal muscles. Patients with a mechanical aortic valve are excluded from implantation of the device because a clot can form on the mechanical prosthesis, which does not open during Novacor LVAD support, and can embolize or occlude the coronary arteries. Because of the extensive implant surgery required, the pump should be implanted before hepatic dysfunction has occurred, as this can contribute to excessive postoperative bleeding. In addition, the patient should have a pre-implantation echocardiogram to rule out a LV apical thrombus, which can complicate implantation.

Implanting the Novacor Pump

The Novacor pump is inserted through a median sternotomy. The incision is extended down to just above the umbilicus. Before the patient is heparinized, a preperitoneal pocket is made on the left, extending just below the costal margin and as far lateral as possible. Similarly, a small preperitoneal pocket is made on the right for the outflow graft to the ascending aorta, but his pocket only need be 2–3 inches wide. After the pockets have been made, the patient is heparinized and cannulated for cardiopulmonary bypass with an arterial cannula in the ascending aorta and two caval cannulas. A PFO should be excluded by either palpation or direct visualization of the atrial septum. The outflow graft from the pump is pre-baked with 25% albumin.

The Novacor pump is placed into the left preperitoneal pocket, and the drive cable is tunneled through the abdominal wall to an exit site just above the right iliac crest. The Dacron outflow graft is anastomosed to the proximal ascending aorta with running 3–0 polypropylene sutures as an end-to-side anastomosis, utilizing a side-biting clamp. The valves are inserted into the pump, and the grafts are connected to the pump. Cardiopulmonary bypass is established, and the heart is kept empty but normothermic and beating. The LV apex is ringed with horizontal pledgetted mattress sutures of 2–0 Ethibond (usually 12). The inflow graft is tunneled through the diaphragm on the left side, just below the costal margin. The left ventricle is elevated and its apex is excised. Clots within the LV apex must be carefully and completely removed to avoid potential embolization. The connection is made between the sewing ring on the apex and the inflow graft. All air is completely removed from the pump, and grafts, and synchronous counterpulsation is begun. The patient is weaned from cardiopulmonary bypass as the Novacor pump takes over the circulation. Bleeding through the insertion site at the LV apex is rare because the left ventricle is totally decompressed. After hemostasis is obtained, the patient is decannulated. The chest and abdomen are closed in the usual fashion with mediastinal drains and a drain in the deepest portion of the left abdominal pocket.

Hemodynamic Management

In our experience at Stanford, the increase in cardiac index and decrease in pulmonary artery diastolic pressure have been quite dramatic following insertion of the Novacor pump (Figure 5). In the early postoperative period, hemodynamic management may be complicated by several factors. First, bleeding may be a problem because of the need for cardiopulmonary bypass and preexisting liver dysfunction. Volume infusion may require multiple procoagulants. In addition, bleeding may lead to tamponade that compresses the left atrium, inhibits filling of the pump, and decreases output.

In addition, right heart dysfunction may not improve immediately, although it can effectively be managed through the liberal use of prostaglandin E_1 (as a pulmonary vasodilator to unload the right ventricle) and inotropic intravenous drips to support RV contractility. Patients with the Novacor pump occasionally require the temporary use of an RV centrifugal pump until pulmonary vascular resistance returns to near normal.

Ventricular arrhythmias occasionally complicate management of the pumps. However, cardiac output has been maintained even in patients who have extended periods of rapid ventricular tachycardia, since LV contraction is not required to fill the pump.

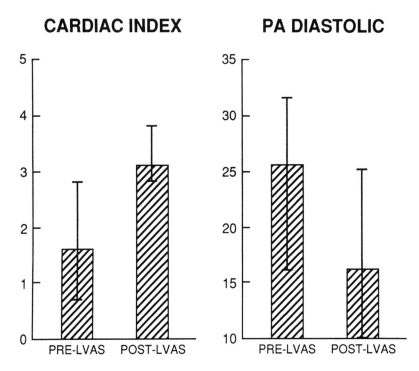

Figure 5. Stanford patients showed significant increases in cardiac index (L/min per m2) and decreases in pulmonary artery (PA) pressure (mmHg) after 24 hours of Novacor support. Reproduced with permission from McCarthy PM, et al. Clinical experience with the Novacor ventricular assist system: Bridge-to-transplant and the transition to chronic application. J Thorac Cardiovasc Surg 1991;102:578–587.

Anticoagulation

An intravenous heparin drip is started as soon as bleeding slows, typically within the first 24 hours. After the patient stabilizes, heparin can be replaced with Coumadin for long-term management. Because of the pericardial tissue valves, the need for long-term anticoagulation is not yet well established, but our current policy is to anticoagulate all patients.

Mobility

One of the major advantages of the wearable Novacor pump over most other circulatory support systems is the high level of activity that the patient can attain after implant surgery. At Stanford, all patients who have had the device for more than a week were walking and sometimes riding stationary bicycles. Such activity is critically important in these patients because they need to regain their strength and stamina before undergoing cardiac transplant. With prolonged support, patients can manage their daily activities and can exercise regularly by using a stationary bicycle and by walking throughout the hospital. To date, patients on the Novacor pump at Stanford have not been transferred to an intermediate discharge facility pending their transplant.

Pump Explant and Heart Transplantation

The longer the pump has been in place, the more extensive the adhesions may be when the patient is ready for transplantation. As a result, we start the transplant operation approximately 60–90 minutes before the anticipated return of the donor heart. The time allows us to mobilize the pump, insert the cannulas, establish bypass, and remove the pump after the grafts have been clamped. The rest of the transplant operation proceeds routinely, except that the anterior ascending aorta (where the outflow graft was inserted from the Novacor pump) must be repaired before the aortic anastomosis can be performed. The pump pocket should be drained.

Results

As of May 1995, 314 patients around the world had received a Novacor bridge-to-transplant pump. This group included 289 men and 25 women, whose mean age was 45 years (range 13–67). One hundred and seventy-four patients had underlying idiopathic cardiomyopathy, 85 had ischemic cardiomyopathy, 31 had acute myocardial infarction, and 24 had other diagnoses (including acute myocarditis and acute allograft rejection). All were in profound heart failure, the mean preimplant cardiac index was 1.90 L/min per m^2 (range 0.7–3.1 L/min per m^2). The mean cardiac index increased to 3.05 L/min per m^2 (range: 1.12–4.56 L/min per m^2) on the Novacor pump. The mean duration of support was 50 days (excluding eight perioperative deaths) and ranged from 1–370 days. Of the 314 patients, 31 were still on support as of May 1995. One hundred and fourteen patients did not survive until transplant (most died of multiorgan failure before transplantation). The remaining 169 patients (60%) underwent cardiac transplant, of whom 156 (92%) were discharged from the hospital. There were 13 early deaths ($\leq$ 1 month) and 13 late ($>$ 1 month) deaths. The overall long-term survival rate was 87%. There have been no mechanical failures of the pump or of the pericardial valves.

Permanent Implantation of the "Wearable" Novacor Pump

Unfortunately, bridging-to-cardiac transplantation fails to solve the shortage of donor organs but merely rearranges the patient priority for transplantation. Following the success of bridging patients to cardiac transplantation for extended periods (> 90 days) using LVADs alone, and the excellent quality of life achieved in most of these patients while waiting for their transplant, the time has arrived to evaluate the wearable Novacor pump as a permanent implant. Preliminary clinical studies have recently commenced in Europe in which the Novacor pump has been placed into patients in whom cardiac transplantation is contraindicated (e.g., too old, excessively elevated pulmonary vascular resistance, unable to tolerate immunosuppressive therapy). These studies will assess the device reliability, patient quality of life, and cost effectiveness of this technology in the management of end-stage cardiac failure.

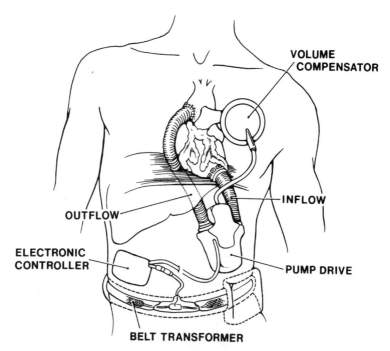

Figure 6. The totally implantable Novacor pump with no percutaneous wires or vents. Reproduced with permission from McCarthy PM, et al. Clinical experience with the Novacor ventricular assist system: Bridge to transplant and the transition to chronic application. J Thorac Cardiovasc Surg 1991;102:578–587.

Totally Implantable Pumps

A totally implantable Novacor pump suitable for long-term use is currently being investigated in animals at Stanford. This system unlike the wearable system has no percutaneous wires or vents, and will be electrically powered with a transcutaneous power source (Figure 6). Offered as an *alternative* to heart transplantation, this system along with the wearable system will help close the gap between donor availability and demand for circulatory support. The present number of heart transplants falls far short of the projected 17,000–30,000 per year who may be acceptable candidates. Many of these patients may be candidates for permanent mechanical LV assistance instead of heart transplantation.

Selected References

1. Bolman RM III, Cox LJ, Marshall W, et al. Circulatory support with a centrifugal pump as a bridge to cardiac transplantation. Ann Thorac Surg 1989;47: 108–112.
2. Golding LAR, Stewart RW, Sinkewich M, et al. Nonpulsatile ventricular assist bridging to transplantation. Trans Am Soc Artif Intern Organs 1988;34:476–479.
3. Gottlieb SO, Brinker JA, Borkon AM, et al. Identification of patients at high risk for vascular complications of intraaortic balloon counterpulsation. Am J Cardiol 1984;53:1135.
4. Farrar DJ. Ventricular interactions during mechanical circulatory support. Semin Thorac Cardiovasc Surg 1994;6:163–168.
5. Frazier OH. Outpatient LVAD: Its time has arrived. Ann Thorac Surg 1994;58: 1309–1310.
6. Frazier OH, Macris MP, Myers TJ, et al. Improved survival after extended bridge to cardiac transplantation. Ann Thorac Surg 1994;57:1416–1422.
7. Karl TR. Extracorporeal circulatory support in infants and children. Semin Thorac Cardiovasc Surg 1994;6:154–160.
8. Kormos RL, Borovetz HS, Gasior T, et al. Experience with univentricular support in mortally ill cardiac transplant candidates. Ann Thorac Surg 1990;49: 261–272.
9. Kormos RL, Murali S, Dew MA, et al. Chronic mechanical circulatory support: Rehabilitation, low morbidity and superior survival. Ann Thorac Surg 1994;57: 51–58.
10. McBride LR. Bridging to cardiac transplantation with external ventricular assist devices. Semin Thorac Cardiovasc Surg 1994;6:169–173.
11. McCarthy PM, Portner PM, Tober HG, et al. Clinical experience with the Novacor ventricular assist system: Bridge-to-transplant and the transition to chronic application. J Thorac Cardiovasc Surg 1991;102:578–587.
12. McCarthy PM, Sabik JF. Implantable circulatory support devices as a bridge to heart transplantation. Semin Thorac Cardiovasc Surg 1994;6:174–180.

13. Magovern GJ, Park SB, Maher TD. Use of a centrifugal pump without anticoagulants for postoperative left ventricular assist. World J Surg 1985;9:25.
14. Oaks TE, Pae WE, Muller CA, et al. Combined registry for the clinical use of mechanical ventricular assist pumps and the total artificial heart in conjunction with heart transplantation: Fifth official report–1990. J Heart Transplant 1991; 10:621–625.
15. Pennington DG, Swartz MT. Mechanical circulatory support prior to cardiac transplantation. Semin Thorac Cardiovasc Surg 1990;2:125–134.
16. Portner PM, Oyer PE, Pennington G, et al. Implantable electrical left ventricular assist system: Bridge to transplantation and the future. Ann Thorac Surg 1989;47:142–150.
17. Reedy JE, Stewart MT, Termuhlen DF, et al. Bridge to heart transplantation: Importance of patient selection. J Heart Transplant 1990;9:473–481.
18. Roberts CP, Wildman D, Woolhouse K, et al. Left ventricular assist with the Biomedicus on a four-month-old infant with anomalous left coronary artery. J Extracorp Tech 1989;21:73–74.
19. Smith JA, Oyer PE, Stinson EB, et al. Bridging to cardiac transplantation with the Novacor left ventricular assist system. Asia Pacific J Thorac Cardiovasc Surg 1994;3:17–24.
20. The Working Group on Mechanical Circulatory Support. Artificial heart and assist device: Directions, needs, costs, societal and ethical issues. Bethesda, Maryland, National Heart, Lung, and Blood Institute, US Department of Health and Human Services, 1985. Report No. (NIH) 85–2723.

Chapter 6

Immunosuppression and Rejection

Patrick M. McCarthy, M.D.,
Margaret E. Billingham, M.D.,
Thomas F. Flavin, M.D., Sharon A. Hunt, M.D.,
Edward B. Stinson, M.D.

Current methods of clinical transplantation are based upon maintaining a balance between immunosuppression, so that responses to the foreign graft are blunted, and infection, so that natural host defenses are not overly impaired. Maintaining this equilibrium is the main responsibility of the transplant physician. It is always in flux. On one hand, when patients are treated with augmented immunosuppression for rejection they may develop serious infection. On the other hand, if life-threatening infections necessitate the reduction of immunosuppression, the risk of rejection subsequently increases. Fortunately, since the clinical introduction of cyclosporine, more specific immunosuppression has become available and the risk of infection has decreased significantly.

Our current 1996 immunosuppression protocol is presented in Table 1. The many consequences of immunosuppression will be covered in Chapters 7 and 8, which discuss infection and other late complications after transplantation. New immunosuppressants soon to be introduced into clinical use will be covered in Chapter 12.

Basic Immunology and Immunosuppression Therapy

The Immunology of Rejection

Ideally, immunosuppression therapy should disarm the immune system in a manner to enable permanent engraftment without compromising host defenses against infection and neoplasia. However, in most instances,

From: Smith JA, McCarthy PM, Sarris GE, Stinson EB, Reitz BA (eds.): The Stanford Manual of Cardiopulmonary Transplantation. Futura Publishing Co., Inc., Armonk, NY, 1996.

Table 1
1996 Clinical Immunosuppression Protocol for Cardiac Transplantation

Immuno-suppression	Pre-op	Intra-op	First 24 hours	Days 1–6	Days 7–14	Maintenance
Cyclosporine	None	None	5–10 mg/kg (divided bid) down nasogastric tube or orally when stable	Adjust to keep level 100–150 ng/mL	Maintain level 150–250 ng/mL	Maintain level 50–150 ng/mL after 30 days
Azathioprine	4 mg/kg IV	None	2 mg/kg IV	2 mg/kg/day IV or orally	2 mg/kg/day	2 mg/kg/day adjust for WBC >5,000/mm$_3$
Methylprednisolone	None	500 mg IV when off cardiopulmonary bypass	125 mg IV Q 8 hours for 3 doses	None	As needed for rejection	As needed for rejection
Prednisone	None	None	None	1.0 mg/kg (divided bid)	If biopsies negative taper after 1 week	0.2 mg/kg/day
OKT3	None	None	Premedicate and give first dose IV drip	Premedicate (days 1–3 only) and IV drip	IV push without premedication days 4–14	As needed for rejection if antibodies to OKT3 are negative

this goal is not possible—there is simply too much overlap between immunologic barriers against foreign tissue (i.e., the allograft) and foreign pathogens. This interaction becomes easier to understand when one considers that the response to antigens from both of these sources occurs in association with the recognition of gene products derived from the major histocompatibility complex (MHC). The activation and proliferation of helper T-lymphocytes (CD4+) are triggered by foreign antigen when it is presented by antigen presenting cells (APC) of the host along with self-MHC Class II gene products. In addition, cytotoxic T-lymphocytes (CD8+ suppressor cells) target cells bearing foreign determinants in association with self-MHC Class I gene products. In transplant patients, the situation is further complicated because MHC products of the donor serve as foreign antigens. Nearly 10- to 100-fold more T-lymphocytes will respond to a given set of MHC alloantigens than respond to non-MHC derived antigens. Thus, the recipient's ability to prevent allograft rejection demands a significant degree of compromise of the patient's immune defense. It is no wonder, then, that the primary cause of death following transplantation is opportunistic infection. Conversely, the current survival rates of most patients are testimony to the dedication and clinical acumen of the transplant physicians, surgeons, and nurses who care for them.

History

Immunosuppression therapy has evolved empirically since the early efforts by Hamburger and co-workers, who used total body irradiation for renal transplantation. The landmark study by Schwartz and Damashek in 1959 demonstrating immunosuppressive properties of 6-mercaptopurine in rabbits prompted Calne, in collaboration with Hitchings and Elion, to evaluate azathioprine (Imuran, Burroughs-Wellcome, Research Triangle Park, NC, USA) for renal transplantation in dogs. This development marked the beginning of clinical pharmacology for immunosuppression. Azathioprine was further evaluated in combination with actinomycin C, azaserine, methotrexate, and trypan blue; however, its combination with prednisone quickly replaced the less effective, more toxic radiotherapy for transplantation in humans.

A more direct assault on the immunoreactive lymphocyte came with the development of xenospecific antisera and antiglobulin terms ALS, ALG, or ATG. These polyclonal antibody preparations were obtained most often by immunizing rabbits or horses with human lymphocytes or thymocytes and absorbing the sera with red cells and hepatocytes to remove irrelevant, potentially harmful cross-reactive antibodies. Borel's discovery of the potent immunosuppressive properties of cyclosporine A (Sandimmune, Sandoz Pharmaceuticals, East Hanover, NJ, USA) in 1976 encouraged Calne to evaluate this agent in several animal models of organ transplantation before he demonstrated its efficacy in clinical trials. Because of its steroid-sparing effects, the widespread use of cyclosporine has resulted in a dramatic decline in the incidence of certain types of opportunistic infections and has made it possible to carry out successful heart-lung transplants.

The development of monoclonal antibodies in 1974 by Kohler and Milstein brought further progress toward more selective alteration of the immune response. These highly specific reagents have contributed enormously to our understanding of the mechanisms responsible for allograft rejection. Monoclonal antibodies permit us to identify subsets of immunoreactive cells involved in the recognition and rejection of foreign tissue. Their clinical utility was first demonstrated in 1981 by Cosimi when, in collaboration with Kung et al, he used the pan T-lymphocyte monoclonal antibody, OKT3 (Ortho Pharmaceutical Corp., Raritan, NJ, USA) to successfully treat acute rejection in patients with kidney transplants. Since then, the immunosuppressive properties of many other monoclonal antibodies directed toward subsets of T-lymphocytes and other cells have been investigated, and preliminary results in rodents and nonhuman primates are promising. The creation of actively acquired tolerance in neonatal animals by Brent, Medawar, and Billingham over 35 years ago stands as the ultimate goal yet to be achieved in the clinical arena.

The Rejection Response

Alloreactive cells recognize highly polymorphic cell surface glycoproteins encoded by the major histocompatibility complex, termed human leukocyte antigen (HLA) in humans (RT in the rat and H-2 in the mouse). Clones of CD4+ helper T-lymphocytes bearing receptors for foreign Class II MHC gene products (HLA, -DR, -D, and -DQ) are activated when presented with these antigens by APCs. Upon activation, these cells proliferate and secrete a variety of soluble polypeptides termed lymphokines. Lymphokines, in turn, recruit other CD4+ T-lymphocytes and initiate a cascade of effector mechanisms, including the differentiation of CD8+ cytoxic T-lymphocytes from precursor cells, antibody secreting plasma cells from B cells, and the migration of natural killer cells and macrophages. Lymphokines such a Il-2, interferon gamma, and tumor necrosis factor alpha induce the expression of Il-2 receptors, MHC Class II gene products, and adhesion molecules such as intercellular adhesion molecule (ICAM)-1. Thus, the consequence of T-lymphocyte activation, whether it occurs within a vascularized organ allograft or in the regional lymph nodes that drain it, is a well orchestrated, focused attack upon the transplant that ultimately results in its rejection.

Immunosuppressants

Cyclosporine

Cyclosporine is a cyclic peptide produced by the fungus *Tolypocladium inflatum gams*. After it was approved by the Food and Drug Administration there was a resurgence of activity in heart, and subsequently in heart-lung and lung transplantation. Unlike cytotoxic immunosuppressants, cyclosporine does not cause myelosuppression. Although its exact mechanism of action is not precisely defined, it selectively inhibits activation of T cells, blocks the release of interleukin-2 from helper T cells, and causes a general reduction in lymphokine release.

For maintenance use, cyclosporine is given orally, usually 6–10 mg/kg per day divided into twice daily doses. Because the drug is oily, it is palatable when mixed with juice, chocolate milk, or milk. The recent introduction of gel-caps may make administration easier and improve patient compliance. Continuous low dose (1–2 mg/kg per day) intravenous cyclosporine infusion is a useful way to initiate therapy immediately after transplantation. The drug can be given intravenously to patients who are incapable of oral administration or have erratic oral absorption, and it can be adjusted according to measured drug levels. In the first 30 days after surgery, we target a trough serum drug level of 200 ng/mL (TDX assay, Abbott Laboratories, North Chicago, IL, USA) and accept levels of 150–250 ng/mL. After 30 days, the level may be allowed to decrease to 100–150 ng/mL.

Trough drug levels (12 hours after last oral dose) vary widely from patient to patient and should be monitored. Peak concentrations are typically observed 3 hours after administration, with most of the drug metabolized by the liver and excreted in the bile. The half-life of cyclosporine is about 6 hours, but it varies widely. Two methods of determining blood concentrations of the drug are widely available: antibody-based radioimmuno-assays (RIA) and high pressure liquid chromatography (HPLC). Whole blood, plasma, or serum may be tested. At Stanford, our standard is an antibody-based, nonisotopic method performed on serum (TDX assay, Abbott Laboratories).

For pediatric patients and cystic fibrosis patients, it is particularly difficult to regulate the cyclosporine dose within the desired therapeutic range.

Pediatric patients may metabolize the drug rapidly and are given TID dosing. Cystic fibrosis patients have erratic absorption and usually receive the drug three times daily with pancreatic enzymes. Doses up to 15–20 mg/kg per day may be required to reach therapeutic levels, and in these cases, the cost of the drug can be very high. In the United States (1992) the approxi-

Table 2
Drug Interactions with Cyclosporine

Drug	Increased CyA Blood Levels	Decreased CyA Blood Levels	Increased Nephrotoxicity
Acetazolamide	*		*
Acyclovir	*		*
Aminoglycoside antibiotics	**		**
Amphotericin B			**
Carbamazepine		**	
Cefotaxime			*
Ceftazidime	*		
Cefuroxime			*
Cephradine			*
Cimetidine	*		**
Ciprofloxacin			*
Danazol	**		*
Diclofenac			*
Digoxin			*
Diltiazem	**		*
Disopyramide			*
Docusate sodium	*		
Doxycycline	**		*
Erythromycin	**		**
Etoposide			*
Ganciclovir			*
Glutethimide		*	
Heparin or ethylenediamine-tetraacetic acid (EDTA)		*	
Imipenem	*		
Indomethacin			*
Isoniazid		**	
Itraconazole	*		*
Josamycin	*		
Ketoconazole	**		**
Levonorgestrel	*		
Macrolides			**
Melphalan	*		
Mesuximide		*	**
Methylprednisolone (high dose therapy)	**		
Methyltestosterone	*		*

mate yearly cost of approximately 6 mg/kg per day of cyclosporine for a 70-kg adult (200-mg bid) is $8,000.

There are many clinically significant drug interactions with cyclosporine that may either increase or decrease clearance and subsequent drug levels. Table 2 contains more complete listing of drug interactions with cyclosporine. Accelerated clearance (decreased levels) is commonly

Table 2 *(continued)*

Drug	Increased CyA Blood Levels	Decreased CyA Blood Levels	Increased Nephrotoxicity
Metoclopramide	**		
Metolazone			*
Metoprolol		*	
Metronidazole	*		
Nafcillin		*	
Nicardipine	**		*
Nifedipine	*		
Nonsterodial anti-inflammatory drugs			*
Norethindrone	*		
Norfloxacin	*		
Octreotide acetate		**	*
Omeprazole (norethisterone)		*	
Oral contraceptives	*		
Phenobarbital		**	
Phenytoin		**	
Prednisolone	**		
Primidone		*	
Pristinamycin	*		*
Ranitidine			**
Rifampin		**	
Sulfadimidine/trimethoprim (IV antibiotic use only)		*	
Sulfamethoxazole	*		
Sulfamethoxazole/trimethoprim (cotrimoxazole)	*		**
Sulfinpyrazone		*	
Tamoxifen	*		
Thiazide diuretics	*		
Ticarcillin	*		
Trimethoprim			**
Valproic acid		*	
Vancomycin			*
Verapamil	**		*
Warfarin	*	*	

* = Suspected/isolated reports (a single documented occurrence of drug interaction)
** = Well substantiated

associated with phenytoin or phenobarbital, rifampin, and intravenous trimethoprim-sulfamethoxazole; the risk of rejection is also higher unless the drug dose is increased. Alternatively, drug toxicity may ensue from decreased clearance (high levels) commonly seen with erythromycin, amphotericin B, ketoconazole, diltiazem, verapamil, danazol, or methylprednisolone. Coadministration of other nephrotoxic drugs (especially aminoglycosides, acyclovir, cotrimoxazole, and melphalan) also may potentiate clinical nephrotoxicity.

The clinical toxicity of cyclosporine primarily involves renal dysfunction, hypertension, neurologic toxicity, and lymphomas. These problems are discussed in Chapters 4 and 8. Hirsutism and gingival hyperplasia are also seen in about 15% of patients treated with cyclosporine. Although not as dangerous as other toxicities, these side effects are very bothersome to some patients.

Corticosteroids

The glucocorticoids (Table 3) act as potent anti-inflammatory agents and immunosuppressants by inhibiting leukocyte elaboration of lymphokines (IL-2 through IL-6), tumor necrosis factor, gamma interferon, granulocyte-macrophage colony-stimulating factor, etc.). Because of their wide-ranging and potent effects, they have had a long history of clinical use in transplantation both for maintenance immunosuppression and treatment of rejection episodes. Our protocol now is to give methylprednisolone early after weaning from cardiopulmonary bypass (500-mg intravenously, then 125 mg every 8 hours for the first 24 hours). When oral medication is started, prednisone is started at 0.6 mg/kg per day (divided into BID doses) and then gradually reduced over 4–6 weeks to 0.2 mg/kg per day. For heart-lung and lung transplant patients, we attempt to withhold steroids (except methylprednisolone) during the first 14 days after

Table 3
Relative Anti-Inflammatory Potency of Corticosteroids

Short-Acting (8–12 hour half-life)		
Cortisol (hydrocortisone)	1	
Intermediate (12–36 hour half-life)		
Prednisone	4	
Methylprednisolone	5	
e.g., 25 mg prednisone	= 31.25 mg methylprednisolone	
	= 6.25 hydrocortisone	

surgery to facilitate healing of the airway anastomosis. In children we try to use every-other-day dosing late in the postoperative period (months) in order to minimize growth retardation. Our success (unlike some other groups) in maintaining patients "steroid-free" long-term has been limited.

Chronic long-term doses of steroids can create many clinical problems, including diabetes, Cushingoid appearance, psychoses, osteoporosis, osteonecrosis, cataracts, skin fragility, hypertension, growth retardation in children, and infections (see Chapters 7 and 8). Therefore, in many programs the trend is to minimize long-term steroids, or withdraw them as early as possible.

Azathioprine

Due to its cytotoxic effects, azathioprine was one of the major clinical immunosuppressants (along with steroids) used before the introduction of cyclosporine. Many transplant centers used cyclosporine and steroids alone during the early 1980s, but most centers added azathioprine (triple drug immunosuppression) by the late 1980s. The bone marrow suppression caused by azathioprine (leukopenia, thrombocytopenia) may be markedly potentiated by allopurinol, and the azathioprine dose must be significantly reduced if allopurinol is used. We usually start with 2 mg/kg per day of azathioprine (either parenteral or enteral) and adjust the dosage in order to get a white blood cell count $> 5,000/mm^3$. The dosage may have to be reduced if viral infection (usually cytomegalovirus [CMV]) causes leukopenia, or if total lymphoid irradiation (TLI) is started.

Murine Monoclonal CD3 Antibody

Murine monoclonal CD3 antibody (OKT3) is the first clinically available monoclonal antibody for immunosuppression. This immunoglobulin, sometimes referred to as a pan T-cell antibody, is directed against the CD3 complex of all T-cells with this receptor. It blocks cellular activation of peripheral lymphocytes.

OKT3 may be used to reverse rejection episodes or prophylactically as induction therapy immediately after transplant surgery. A reported "first-dose" response (chills, fever, dyspnea, wheezing, tremor, pulmonary edema) may be due to lymphokine release from the affected T-cells. To minimize this problem, at Stanford, the first three doses of OKT3 are infused over 1 hour (rather than "push"), and anti-inflammatory prophylaxis

Table 4
OKT3 Administration Protocol

Days 1–3
  1. Premedication (at 1600 hours daily for 3 days).
      Tylenol 650 mg by mouth or rectally
      Ranitidine 100 mg IV
      Benadryl 25 mg IV
      Hydrocortisone 100 mg IV
  2. Then give OKT3 5 mg (1 amp) in 50 cc 5% dextrose and water. Run over 1
     hour. Start infusion at 1630 hours every day for 3 days.
  3. Continue every 6 hours for 3 days, then discontinue.
      Tylenol 650 mg by mouth or rectally
      Ranitidine 50 mg IV
Days 4–14
  1. No premedication.
  2. OKT3 5 mg (1 amp) IV push daily for 11 days.

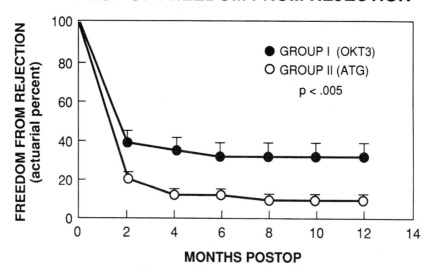

Figure 1. Fewer rejection episodes were seen in Stanford patients given OKT3 induction vs rATG induction. Reproduced with permission from Starnes VA, et al. Circulation 1989;80(Suppl III):III-79-III-83.

is given before the doses are administered (Table 4). Anti-idiotypic anti-bodies (to the murine portion of the immunoglobulin) develop in ap-proximately 15% of patients and limit retreatment for later rejection episodes in this subgroup. When compared to our previous patients treated with polyclonal antithymocyte globulins (rabbit ATG), OKT3 treated pa-tients had significantly fewer rejection episodes (Figure 1) and similar rates of infection and overall survival. Others, however, have found similar effi-cacy in randomized studies. In our recently updated experience of heart transplantation in the cyclosporine era, the patients treated with induction OKT3 had reduced early linearized rejection rates and prolonged time to first rejection although long-term, there was no difference in terms of free-dom from rejection, infection and in overall survival. During treatment with OKT3, T-lymphocyte counts should be monitored in order to docu-ment at least one aspect of biological effectiveness. Generally, we aim for T-cell counts around 1% or an absolute count of $< 200/mm^3$ (normal 680–2,480), as measured by FACS analysis.

Clinical Manifestations of Cardiac Rejection

Cardiac rejection may be asymptomatic and detected by routine en-domyocardial biopsy, or it may present as a rapidly progressive, dramatic, fatal event. Although rejection is most often seen within the first 3 months after transplantation, it may occur at any time, even years later.

The clinical clues to rejection are nonspecific and include fatigue, malaise, dyspnea, and anorexia. Fever may be present as well as edema, hy-pertension (absolute or relative), jugular venous distention, abnormal heart sounds, and friction rub. A more subtle clue to rejection is frequently seen in a patient being treated for hypertension. Because of brief episodes of relative hypotension, the antihypertensive medications are withheld and the patient becomes normotensive. Another clinical clue is supraventricular arrhyth-mias; these are relatively specific for rejection, especially if they begin 2–4 weeks after transplant surgery. An occasional severe rejection episode will progress to hemodynamic instability, and the patient will present with the clinical picture of cardiogenic shock. These clinical signs and symptoms may herald a rejection episode, and we recommend proceeding promptly with en-domyocardial biopsy, even though there may be another explantation.

Noninvasive methods of detecting rejection are not yet specific and sensitive enough for routine clinical use. The previously useful electrocar-diographic criterion for rejection (decreased voltage in the QRS complex) became unreliable after the introduction of cyclosporine. Investigations of echocardiographic and Doppler indices of diastolic left ventricular dys-function are promising methods that show good correlation with histologic changes, but they are not used alone as a guide to anti-rejection therapy. Many other noninvasive methods of detecting functional changes are being investigated (e.g., magnetic resonance imaging, thallium-201 imaging, wall motion analysis by myocardial markers), but none of these are clinically useful as yet. Right ventricular endomyocardial biopsy remains the gold standard against which other methods are compared.

Monitoring Acute Rejection by Endomyocardial Biopsies in Heart and Combined Heart-Lung Transplant Recipients

Techniques of Right Ventricular Endomyocardial Biopsy

The purposes of endomyocardial biopsy in managing heart and heart-lung recipients are to: 1. diagnose acute rejection; 2. assess the results of treatment for acute rejection; 3. diagnose infectious myocarditis (usually CMV or toxoplasmosis); and 4. assess myocardial ischemia immediately after transplantation. The routine schedule of endomyocardial biopsy after transplantation is as follows:

1. Every week for the first 6 weeks, then,
2. Every other week until 3 months, then,
3. Every month until 6 months, then,
4. Every 3 months.

Biopsies are also repeated approximately 1 week after an episode of treated rejection in order to document resolution. In a patient with a record of multiple rejection episodes, biopsies are performed more frequently.

Sampling error is inherent in endomyocardial biopsy, therefore, it is essential that a minimum of three good pieces of myocardium be obtained using a 9 Fr bioptome to reduce sampling error. If a small French bioptome is used, more pieces are needed. Biopsies on infants and children also require more pieces of myocardium. The procedure is performed under local anesthesia, usually with oral premedication. The preferred approach is via the right internal jugular vein, but the left internal jugular vein, either subclavian vein, or either femoral vein may be used if necessary. The femoral approach is preferred for infants and small children. At Stanford, fluoroscopy has been routinely used to guide the bioptome (either in the cardiac catheterization lab or in the operating room with a portable system), but at other institutions and more recently at Stanford, echocardiography has been used successfully for this purpose.

After the neck and upper chest have been prepped and draped, the vein is punctured and a wire introduced using the Seldinger technique. An introducer sheath with a one-way valve is passed into the vein. The Cave's bioptome (9 Fr for adults, 7 Fr for children) is advanced into the right atrium under fluoroscopic visualization (Figure 2). The bioptome is ro-

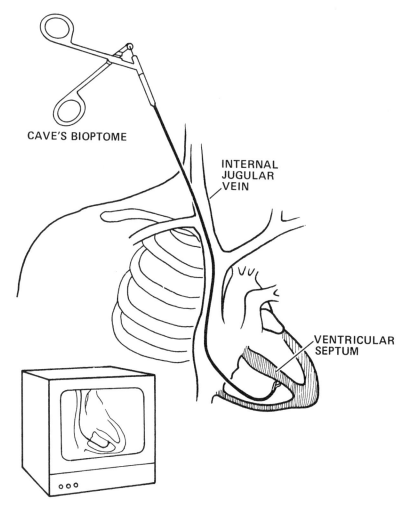

Figure 2. Endomyocardial biopsy of the right ventricular septum via the right internal jugular vein using fluoroscopy and continuous ECG monitoring.

tated 90° and advanced across the tricuspid valve into the right ventricle. This turn is sometimes difficult because the right atrial suture line along the atrial septum may "catch" the bioptome. The bioptome is rotated another 90° to direct it into the septum and away from the ventricular free wall. Electrocardiographic monitoring is important, as short runs or premature ventricular contractions are common, and ventricular tachycardia or fibrillation are possible consequences. Typically, 4–6 acceptable pieces (1–2 mm) of myocardium are taken and sent for processing. The bioptome and introducer are then removed, and the patient's hemodynamic status is closely monitored for 1 hour after biopsy. In over 2,000 biopsies at Stanford, there has been only one fatal ventricular perforation, in a neonate who was undergoing biopsy for acute rejection.

Processing of Endomyocardial Biopsy

The biopsy pieces should be fixed immediately in 10% buffered formalin, labeled correctly, and sent to the pathology laboratory for processing. Following adequate fixation, these biopsies are processed in the usual way of dehydration and paraffin embedding. The following rules should be adhered to:

1. All sections should be under 4 μ in thickness (thicker sections will result in erroneous results).
2. All pieces of biopsy may be embedded in the same block, but they should be carefully counted to make sure all are present.
3. The paraffin block should be cut all the way through in "step" sections, and the sections should be stained routinely with hematoxylin and eosin and a connective tissue stain (Masson's trichrome stain). Methyl green pyronine stain to highlight activated lymphocytes is optional.
4. If immunohistochemistry for lymphocyte subset markers is to be used, then a fragment of tissue should be snap frozen at the time of the biopsy. Electron microscopy is not useful for routine surveillance of rejection.

If the biopsy is required urgently, the pathologist should be informed and "ultra" processing should be used. Fixation and processing in this technique are similar to those described above, except that a vacuum infiltrating technicon processor is used to process the tissue in 90 minutes instead of the 10-hour cycle. A permanent section is obtained from the "ultra" method, and the sections are stained in the usual way.

Occasionally, in an extreme emergency, it is necessary to perform a frozen section on a biopsy specimen. The tissue is frozen, mounted in freezing mixture on a cryostat chuck, and then cut into thin sections as for other frozen sections. Stains should be with hematoxylin and eosin. If preferred and if an adequate number of pieces are available, one piece of tissue may be frozen for immunohistochemical studies. The specimen is placed in a plastic Beem capsule filled with freezing mixture and immersed in liquid nitrogen or isopentane and dry ice. Tissue may then be stored indefinitely at $-70°C$. Except for special research studies, we do not routinely culture endomyocardial biopsy specimens.

Histopathological Changes in the Early Post Period Transplantation

Hyperacute Rejection

Hyperacute rejection usually manifests itself immediately while the patient is in the operating room, and an endomyocardial biopsy diagnosis is not usually required. For the sake of completeness, the histopathologic changes, will be briefly described. Marked interstitial edema and diffuse hemorrhage are noted throughout the myocardium. Small vessels may contain fibrin thrombi and "sludging" of red cells. The initial biopsy within 24 hours after cardiac transplantation may show hyperacute rejection, although this is very rare.

Reperfusion and Ischemic Injury

The first biopsies following cardiac transplantation are usually performed at or within 1 week of the procedure. Ischemic changes are seen that result from prolonged preservation of the donor heart or extended operative time. Microscopically, areas of early myocytolysis and coagulation of the myocyte cytoplasm (which may be highlighted by a gray color when stained with Masson's trichrome) may be seen with little or no inflammatory infiltrate. The amount of myocyte damage is usually more than that seen in moderate acute rejection. Although myocyte contraction bands are often seen as well as hypereosinophilia, these may occur as an artifact in the biopsy; therefore, this sign is not useful. Focal ischemic patches, even if diffuse, do not usually require any treatment. Very rarely, inadvertent surgical trauma at the time of cardiac transplantation will result in a myocardial infarction of the donor heart. It may be difficult to separate infarct from is-chemic reperfusion injury; however, necrotic myocardium and neutro-philic infiltrate may be seen in the case of infarcts.

Myocardial Damage Due to Pressor Agents

Sympathomimetic pressor agents may have been used before harvesting to support the donor heart or after cardiac transplantation to support the re-cipient. If enough of these agents are used, focal areas of myocyte necrosis with sparse mixed inflammatory infiltrate may be seen, which is typical of the catecholamine effect. A small area of focal myocardial injury with a mixed in-filtrate in the first week should not be confused with acute rejection.

Microinfarcts

In the first and second endomyocardial biopsies following cardiac transplantation, small microinfarcts are often seen appearing as focal myo-cyte damage without lymphocytic infiltrates. The microinfarcts are thought to be due to trapped air bubbles within the coronary circulation at the time of reperfusion of the transplanted heart. Masson's trichrome is useful to highlight these areas.

Acute Rejection

Although uncommon, acute rejection may occur within the first 10 days after cardiac transplantation, depending on the degree of histocom-patibility mismatching between donor and recipient and also on the type of prophylactic immunosuppression used. Acute rejection can be distin-guished from ischemia because lymphocytic infiltrate is always greater than myocyte damage in rejection, while the reverse is true in ischemia. Table 5 summarizes the Stanford grading system, as described previously.

Mild Acute Rejection

Mild acute rejection is manifested by an early perivascular mononuclear inflammatory infiltrate of pyroninophilic lymphocytes (Figure 3). These ac-tivated lymphocytes are dark, large, and round and may have prominent nu-cleoli. The earliest manifestation is localization in a perivascular distribution,

Table 5
Morphologic Grading of Acute Rejection (Stanford)

Grade of Rejection	Morphologic Features
Mild acute rejection	Sparse perivascular, endocardial, or interstitial infiltrate by activated lymphocytes
Moderate acute rejection	Focal or more diffuse patchy infiltrate of activated lymphocytes and eosinophils surrounding myocytes and often causing focal damage
Severe acute rejection	Florid infiltrate of activated lymphocytes, eosinophils, and neutrophils with vasculitis and hemorrhage
Resolving acute rejection	Lymphocytes are fewer and smaller (inactivated)— Reparative changes of fibrous scar and hemosiderin-laden macrophages

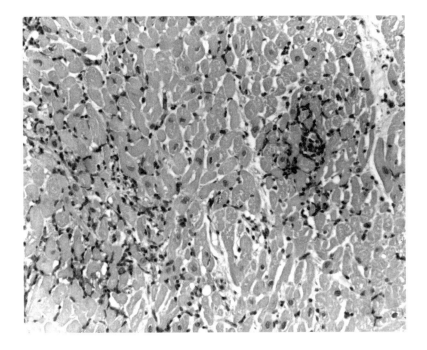

Figure 3. Cardiac biopsy showing a scanty infiltrate of lymphocytes without myocyte damage, indicating mild acute rejection. Hematoxylin and eosin, original magnification × 160.

but the lymphocyte may also be present focally in the endocardial surface or the interstitium. Myocyte damage is usually not present. The spectrum of mild acute rejection ranges from a focal perivascular infiltrate or focal interstitial infiltrate in one piece of tissue to a sparse interstitial infiltrate in two or more pieces, but without myocyte damage. Mild acute rejection does not require augmentation of immunosuppression therapy at Stanford. However, this diagnosis is important for three reasons:

1. It should alert the clinician to an impending episode of acute rejection requiring treatment;
2. In the case of patients transplanted before the advent of cyclosporine and maintained on conventional therapy with prednisone and azathioprine alone, treatment was instituted immediately as such patients can develop acute rejection much more rapidly (this may also apply to patients in whom cyclosporine has been discontinued);
3. Approximately 40%–50% of episodes of mild acute rejection in cyclosporine-treated patients proceed to moderate acute rejection on a follow-up biopsy within 1 week. Patients, therefore, routinely receive a biopsy 5–7 days following a diagnosis of mild acute rejection.

Moderate Acute Rejection

Moderate acute rejection occurs when the lymphocytic infiltrate in the biopsy extends into the interstitium in several of the pieces submitted for examination (Figure 4). Plump activated lymphocytes may line up along the margins of myocytes or completely surround them, causing indentation and actual necrosis. In most patients with moderate acute rejection the infiltrate is a monomorphous lymphocytic one, although in cyclosporine-treated patients, the presence of eosinophils is not unusual. If a moderate inflammatory infiltrate is present in two or three pieces of tissue, a diagnosis of moderate acute rejection should be made in our opinion even if myocyte damage is minimal. The spectrum of moderate acute rejection ranges from a definite infiltrate with focal necrosis in one or two pieces to a fairly extensive interstitial infiltrate of activated lymphocytes, but without neutrophils and hemorrhage.

Severe Acute Rejection

In severe acute rejection, the inflammatory infiltrate becomes much more marked and is usually present in every piece of the endomyocardial

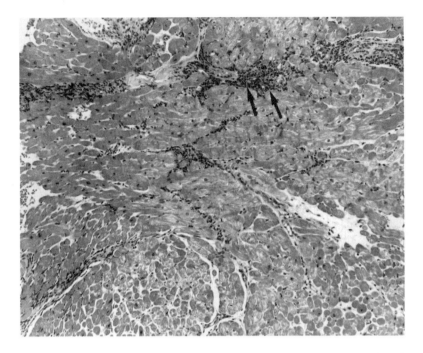

Figure 4. Cardiac biopsy showing perivascular lymphocytic infiltrates extending into the interstitium and causing focal myocyte damage (arrows) and replacement (moderate acute rejection). Hematoxylin and eosin, original magnification × 160.

biopsy. At this stage there may be vasculitides (Figure 5), resulting in interstitial hemorrhage, and the inflammatory infiltrate is often mixed, not only with eosinophils, but also with neutrophils. The presence of a mixed inflammatory infiltrate should also alert the pathologist to rule out infectious myocarditis. With cyclosporine-treated patients, the neutrophilic infiltrate is not as marked as in conventionally-treated patients. Edema may or may not be present although it is difficult to distinguish edema from artifact in an endomyocardial biopsy. Whatever treatment regimen is being applied whenever there is severe acute rejection, rapid augmentation of immunosuppression is mandatory if the patient is to be saved. It is easier to reverse severe acute rejection in cyclosporine-treated patients than in conventionally-treated patients.

Resolving or Resolved Acute Rejection

After successful treatment of acute rejection, the subsequent biopsy may show a reduced number of activated lymphocytes in the interstitium, together

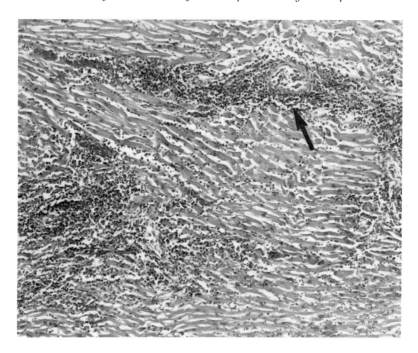

Figure 5. Cardiac biopsy showing a more diffuse infiltrate, vasculitis (arrow), and hemorrhage (severe acute rejection). Hematoxylin and eosin, original and magnification × 160.

with reparative changes of early fibrosis and hemosiderin-laden macrophages. If a small number of active lymphocytes remain at the time of a follow-up biopsy, a diagnosis of resolving acute rejection is usually made; however, if the biopsy contains only scattered nonactivated lymphocytes with early scar formation, then a diagnosis of resolved acute rejection can be made.

Pitfalls of Diagnosing Acute Rejection by Endomyocardial Biopsy

Inadequate Tissue

The most common pitfall for the diagnosis of acute rejection by endomyocardial biopsy is insufficient tissue. Sampling error is inherent in the endomyocardial biopsy procedure; therefore, three to four pieces of tissue with a 9 Fr bioptome should be available for screening. Occasionally, biopsies consist also of thrombus, blood clot, or adipose tissue from the subepicardium. In the case of subepicardial adipose tissue, an inflammatory infiltrate resulting from the operative procedure may be present, but this infiltrate should not be interpreted as acute rejection unless it extends into the myocardium, particularly within the first 2 or 3 weeks after cardiac transplantation. If the adipose tissue contains mesothelial cells, the clinician should be warned that ventricular perforation may have taken place.

Previous Biopsy Sites

Cardiac transplant recipients have many serial endomyocardial biopsies, and recipients have had between 30 and 50 procedures. Because several pieces of tissue are taken at each procedure, many biopsies include a previous biopsy site. The pathologist should distinguish a recent biopsy site that contains fibrin and granulation tissue from acute rejection. If the biopsy site has begun to heal, myocyte disarray at the base of the site is a useful marker to distinguish it from a focus of acute rejection. Older biopsy sites show fibrosis, myocyte disarray, and thickened endocardium. Occasionally, lymphocytic infiltrates are trapped in the biopsy site.

Endocardial Infiltrates ("Quilty" Effect)

Since the use of cyclosporine-based immunosuppression for cardiac allograft recipients, focal endocardial infiltrates of pyroninophilic lymphocytes ("Quilty" effect) have been present in approximately 9% of all endomyocardial biopsies in the Stanford series. In general, these infiltrates are confined to the endocardium and are above the endocardial surface, although occasional spillover into the subjacent myocardium can be seen. They have also been reported to be associated with some myocyte damage. Although these infiltrates may be a part of the rejection process, they do not necessarily disappear with increased immunosuppression. It has been our policy at Stanford not to treat these "Quilty" effects.

Infectious Myocarditis

In any immunosuppressed patient, the possibility of infectious myocarditis is always present, particularly that of CMV and *Toxoplasma gondii*. The pathologist should be alerted when a donor heart from a CMV-seropositive patient is placed in a CMV-seronegative recipient, and close liaison with the transplant team should be maintained so that information about rising serum titers is available. Sometimes it is difficult not to distinguish an inflammatory infiltrate due to infectious myocarditis from that of acute rejection. The inflammatory infiltrate of CMV myocarditis is a mixed infiltrate with more eosinophils than are usually seen in acute rejection; more myocyte damage is also present. Whenever there is a mixed inflammatory infiltrate, the pathologist should always look for and rule out either CMV or toxoplasma infection; DNA probes can be used for the former. Also, if the toxoplasma cysts are still intact, an inflammatory infiltrate may not be evoked. Occasionally, CMV inclusions may be seen in myocyte nuclei that are surrounded only by edema and not by an inflammatory infiltrate. It is possible to have both rejection and infection at the same time, and, if that occurs, the patient is usually treated for infection rather than for rejection insofar as possible. Other infections caused by fungi such as Aspergillus, Candida, Blastomyces, or Coccidioides can also be detected by an endomyocardial biopsy. A mixed inflammatory infiltrate that included eosinophils in an endomyocardial biopsy should always require thorough search of all biopsy pieces at all levels to rule out infection.

Grading of Acute Cardiac Rejection

Several different grading systems for acute cardiac rejection are now in use and each center should use the one it prefers and is most familiar with. In any one center, however, the grading system should remain consistent to avoid confusion in patient management. The main grading systems previously used to describe acute rejection are listed in Table 6. The current "universal" grading system standardized under the auspices of the International Society for Heart Transplantation is presented in Table 7.

Table 6
Grading Systems for Active Rejection

System	Grading
Standford Grading System (Billingham)	3 major grades + "Resolving" rejection
Texas Grading System (McAllister)	10 major grades
Hannover Grading System (Kemnitz)	5 major grades + "Chronic" rejection
Pittsburgh Grading System (Zerbe)	4 major grades
Brigham Grading System (Schoen)	7 major grades
Boston Consortium Grading System (Schoen)	5 major grades

Table 7
ISHT Standardized Cardiac Biopsy Grading

Grade	New Nomenclature	Old Nomenclature
0	No rejection	No rejection
1	A—Focal (perivascular or interstitial) infiltrate without necrosis	Mild rejection
	B—Diffuse but sparse infiltrate without necrosis	
2	One focus only with aggressive infiltration	"Focal" moderate rejection
3	A—Multifocal aggressive infiltrates and/or myocyte damage	"Low" moderate rejection
	B—Diffuse inflammatory process with necrosis	"Borderline/severe"
4	Diffuse aggressive polymorphous ± infiltrate ± edema, ± hemorrhage, ± vasculitis, with necrosis	

Reproduced with permission from Billingham ME, Carey NRB, Hammond ME, et al. A working formulation for the standardization of nomenclature in the diagnosis of heart and lung rejection: Heart rejection study group. J Heart Transplant 1990; 9:587–593.

Treatment of Cardiac Rejection

First Rejection Episode

Histologically mild rejection is not treated with augmented immunosuppression unless it is unduly persistent. The patient is carefully followed and repeat biopsies are performed to evaluate the patient's progress. Moderate or severe rejection episodes are treated, and the patient is admitted to the intensive care unit if there are hemodynamic changes. Early rejection after transplantation is treated with a pulse of steroids (methylprednisolone 1-gm intravenously per day for 3 days). Children are treated with 10–15 mg/kg of methylprednisolone per dose. Moderate episodes of rejection without hemodynamic changes, as detected by routine surveillance biopsy, can be treated safely on an outpatient basis with increased oral steroids (prednisone 100 mg BID for 3 days). Approximately 80% of rejection episodes will resolve with pulsed steroids as determined by follow-up endomyocardial biopsy.

Ongoing and Repeated Rejection

Further episodes of rejection (with intervening resolving, mild, or negative biopsies since the previous episode) are usually treated with another pulse of steroids. Ongoing rejection, especially if severe, is treated with more intensive immunosuppression. If this episode is so late (> 1 month) that antibody titers to OKT3 have been measured and found to be negative (< 1:100), then a second course of OKT3 (10–14 days) may be used. If significant antimurine antibody titers exist (10%–15% of patients), repeated OKT3 treatment may still be effective if dosages are augmented sufficiently to produce antibody excess and thereby depress measured T-lymphocyte counts to targeted levels. There is a risk, however, of severe allergic reactions. Alternatively, a relatively short (3–5 days) course of rabbit antithymocyte globulin (rATG) may be given. Several such preparations have proven efficacious in reversing acute cardiac rejection. Their disadvantages are the lack of commercial availability and uncertain variation in potency. As expected, antibody formation to rabbit protein may also occur and may produce allergic reactions, including serum sickness, as well as limit repetitive administration. However, for most patients with ongoing moderate rejection and no hemodynamic changes, another pulse of methylprednisolone is given before proceeding with rATG or repeat OKT3.

Rarely patients continue to have rejection or have multiple episodes over a period of weeks, despite pulsed steroids and rATG or OKT3. Limited clinical use of TLI (up to 800 cGy total; 80 cGy per treatment, 2 times per week) appears quite promising. Azathioprine must be sharply decreased or stopped before TLI begins because the white blood cell count falls rapidly. TLI is usually withheld if the count falls below 2,000 WBC/mm^3. Thrombocytopenia may also necessitate interruption of treatment. During the course of irradiation, T-lymphocyte counts and subset analyses are followed; profound depression of total lymphocyte and both CD4+ and CD8+ counts occurs promptly and may last for several months.

Overall, our published experience with TLI for intractable acute rejection includes 10 patients who received 240–800 cGy each over 2–24 weeks. In all patients rejection resolved as shown by biopsy 2–4 weeks after treatment was started. Seven patients subsequently sustained recurrent rejection episodes 40–769 days after TLI, but these episodes were generally easily controlled. Further, after TLI, 90% of patients could be maintained on lower maintenance doses of prednisone. Despite the somewhat cumbersome details involved in the use of TLI, it is a very useful technique in the management of selected patients with recurrent graft rejection.

Very rarely, patients continue to have rejection episodes despite all treatment and are considered for retransplantation. By this point, however, patients are profoundly immunosuppressed. Many will have developed opportunistic infection or other complications, and most patients are no longer retransplant candidates. Results of retransplantation for intractable acute rejection are disappointing; in our experience with 17 such cases, 1-year survival was only 33%.

Selected References

1. Alexandre GPJ, Murray JE. Further studies of renal homotransplantation in dogs treated by combined immuran therapy. Surg Forum 1962;13:64–66.
2. Beato M. Gene regulation by steroid hormones. Cell 1989;56:315–344.
3. Billingham ME. Diagnosis of cardiac rejection by endomyocardial biopsy. Heart Transplant 1982;1:25.
4. Billingham ME. Cardiac transplantation. Cardiovasc Clin 1988;18:185–199.
5. Billingham ME. The postsurgical heart. Am J Cardiovasc Pathol 1988;1:319–334.
6. Billingham ME, Carey NRB, Hammond ME, et al. A working formulation for the standardization of nomenclature in the diagnosis of heart and lung rejection: Heart rejection study group. J Heart Transplant 1990;9:587–593.
7. Billingham ME, Krohn PL, Medawar PB. Effect locally applied cortisone acetate on survival of skin homografts in rabbits. Br Med J 1951;2:1049.
8. Borel JF, Feurer C, Magnee C, et al. Effects of the new anti-lymphocytic peptide cyclosporine A in animals. Immunology 1977;32:1017–1025.
9. Bristow MR, Renlund DG, Gilbert EM, et al. Murine monoclonal CD-3 antibody in cardiac transplantation: Antirejection treatment and preliminary results in a prospectively randomized trial for prophylaxis. Clin Transplant 1988;2:163–168.
10. Calne RY. Rejection of renal homografts: Inhibition in dogs by 6-Mercaptopurine. Lancet 1960;1:417–418.
11. Calne RY. Immunosuppression for organ grafting—observations on cyclosporin A. Immunolog Rev 1979;46:113–124.
12. Dupont E. Molecular and cellular mechanisms of action of drugs used to modulate the immune response. Semin Thorac Cardiovasc Surg 1990;2:175–180.
13. Elion GB. The purine path to chemotherapy. Science 1989;244:41–47.
14. Frist WH, Oyer PE, Baldwin JC, et al. HLA compatibility and cardiac transplant recipient survival. Ann Thorac Surg 1987;44:242–246.
15. Frist WH, Winterland AQ, Gerhardt EB, et al. Total lymphoid irradiation in heart transplantation: Adjunctive treatment for recurrent rejection. Ann Thorac Surg 1989;48:863–864.
16. Grattan MT, Moreno-Cabral CE, Starnes VA, et al. Eight-year results of cyclosporine-treated patients with cardiac transplants. J Thorac Cardiovasc Surg 1990;99:500–509.
17. Greene PS, Cameron DE, Augustine S, et al. Exploratory analysis of time-dependent risk for infection, rejection, and death after cardiac transplantation. Ann Thorac Surg 1989;47:650–654.
18. Hakim M, Wallwork J, English T. Cyclosporin A in cardiac transplantation: Medium-term results in 62 patients. Ann Thorac Surg 1988;46:495–501.
19. Hamburger J, Vaysse J, Crosnier J, et al. Renal homotransplantation in man after radiation of the recipient: Experience with six patients since 1959. Am J Med 1962;32:854–871.
20. Handschumacher RE. Immunosuppressive agents. In: Gilman A, ed. The Phar-

macological Basis of Therapeutics. Eighth Edition. Elmsford, NY, Pergamon Press, 1990, pp. 1264–1276.
21. Haynes RC Jr. Adrenocorticotropic hormone; adrenocortical steroids and their synthetic analogs; inhibitors of the synthesis and actions of adrenocortical hormones. In: Gilman A, ed. The Pharmacological Basis of Therapeutics. Eighth Edition. Elmsford, NY, Pergamon Press, 1990, pp. 1431–1462.
22. Hunt SA. Clinical and non-invasive methods of monitoring rejection. In: Gallucci V, ed. Heart and Heart-Lung Transplantation Update. Firenze, Italy, Uses Edizioni Scientifiche, 1988, pp. 107–109.
23. Jacquet L, Ziady G, Stein K, et al. Cardiac rhythm disturbances early after orthotopic heart transplantation: Prevalence and clinical importance of the observed abnormalities. J Am Coll Cardiol 1990;16:832–837.
24. Kemnitz J, Cohnert T, Schafers H-J, et al. A classification of cardiac allograft rejection. Am J Surg Pathol 1987;7:503.
25. Kung PC, Goldstein G, Reinherz EL, et al. Monoclonal antibodies defining distinctive human T cell surface antigens. Science 1979;206:347–349.
26. Krensky AM, Weiss A, Crabtree G, et al. T-lymphocyte-antigen interactions in transplant rejection. N Engl J Med 1990;322(8):510–517.
27. Lake KD. Cyclosporine drug interactions: A review. In: Cardiac Surgery State of the Art Reviews. Vol. 2, No. 4. Philadelphia, Hanley & Belfus, Inc, 1988, pp. 617–630.
28. Liem BL, DiBiase A, Schroeder JS. Arrhythmias and clinical electrophysiology of the transplanted human heart. Semin Thorac Cardiovasc Surg 1990;2:271–278.
29. McAllister HA, Schree MJ, Radovanceivc B, et al. A system for grading cardiac allograft rejection. Texas Heart Inst J 1986;13:1.
30. Modry DL, Strober S, Hoppe RT. Total lymphoid irradiation: Experimental models and clinical application in organ transplantation. Heart Transplant 1983;2:122–135.
31. Murray JE, Merrill JP, Harrison JH, et al. Prolonged survival of human-kidney homografts by immunosuppressive drug therapy. N Engl J Med 1963;268:1320–1323.
32. Nakatani T, Aida H, Frazier OH, et al. Effect of ABO blood type on survival of heart transplant patients treated with cyclosporine. J Heart Transplant 1989;8:27–33.
33. Renlund DG, O'Connell JB, Gilbert EM, et al. A prospective comparison of murine monoclonal CD3 (OKT3) antibody based and equine antithymocyte globulin based rejection prophylaxis in cardiac transplantation: Decreased rejection/less corticosteroid use with OKT3. Transplantation 1989;47:599–605.
34. Renlund DG, O'Connell JB, Bristow MR. Strategies of immunosuppression in cardiac transplantation. Semin Thorac Cardiovasc Surg 1990;2:181–188.
35. Rose ML, Yacoub M. Mechanisms of cardiac allograft rejection and avenues for immunological monitoring. Semin Thorac Cardiovasc Surg 1990;2:162–174.
36. Russell PS, Colvin RB, Cosimi AB. Monoclonal antibodies for the diagnosis and treatment of transplant rejection. Ann Rev Med 1984;35:63–79.
37. Sarris GE, Moore KA, Schroeder JS, et al. Cardiac transplantation: The Stanford experience in the cyclosporine era. J Thorac Cardiovasc Surg 1994:108:240–251.
38. Schoen FJ, ed. Interventional and Surgical Cardiovascular Pathology. Philadelphia, WB Saunders, 1989, p. 195.

39. Schwartz R, Damashek W. Drug induced immunologic tolerance. Nature 1959; 183:1682.
40. Smith JA, Ribakove GH, Hunt SA, et al. Heart retransplantation: The 25 year experience at a single institution. J Heart Lung Transplant 1995;14:832–839.
41. Starnes VA, Oyer PE, Stinson EB, et al. Prophylactic OKT3 used as induction therapy for heart transplantation. Circulation 1989;80(Suppl III):III-79-III-83.
42. Starzl TE, Iwatsuki S, Van Thiel DH, et al. Evolution of liver transplantation. Hepatology 1982;2:614–636.
43. Starzl TE, Marchioro TL, Porter KA, et al. The use of heterologous antilymphoid agents in canine renal and liver homotransplantation and in human renal homotransplantation. Surg Gynecol Obstet 1967;124(2):301–308.
44. Strober S, Dhillon M, Schubert M, et al. Acquired immune tolerance to cadaveric renal allografts. A study of three patients treated with total lymphoid irradiation. N Engl J Med 1989;321:28–33.
45. Sweeney MC, Macris MP, Frazier OH, et al. The treatment of advanced cardiac allograft rejection. Ann Thorac Surg 1988;46:378–381.
46. Takahashi N, Hayano T, Suzuki M. Peptidyl-prolyl Cis-trans isomerase in the cyclosporine A-binding protein cyclophilin. Nature 1989;337:473–475.
47. Wahlers T, Heublein B, Cremer J, et al. Treatment of rejection after heart transplantation: What dosage of pulsed steroids is necessary? J Heart Transplant 1990;9:568–574.
48. Zerbe TR, Arena V. Diagnostic reliability of endomyocardial biopsy for assessment of cardiac allograft rejection. Human Pathol 1988;19:1307–1313.
49. Zukoski CF, Lee HM, Hume DRM. Prolongation of functional survival of canine renal homografts by 6-Mercaptopurine. Surg Forum 1960;11:470–472.

Chapter 7

Surveillance and Treatment of Posttransplant Infections

Anne M. Keogh, M.B., B.S., M.D., FRACP,
Sharon A. Hunt, M.D., Patricia Gamberg, R.N.,
Edward B. Stinson, M.D.

The use of cyclosporine-based immunosuppression after cardiac transplantation (see Chapter 6) has led to a reduction in deaths from infectious complications (particularly fungal), as compared with conventional immunosuppression using prednisone and azathioprine only. However, infection remains the leading cause of death following cardiac transplantation; in the Stanford series, infection accounted for 34% of all deaths during the cyclosporine era since December 1980. Infection is most likely to occur in the first year after transplantation, particularly in the weeks immediately after transplant surgery and after augmentation of immunosuppression for rejection. Depending on a patient's rejection history, reducing the overall level of immunosuppression may be possible and even necessary as an adjunct to appropriate antibiotic therapy during life-threatening infections. In the Stanford series, bacterial infections accounted for 48% of infectious episodes after transplantation, viral for 32%, fungal 10%, protozoan 6%, and nocardia for 4% (Tables 1 and 2). Mixed infections are common.

We recommend standard antibiotic prophylaxis for cardiac transplant recipients undergoing dental procedures and gastrointestinal or genitourinary tract surgery because of the possibility of developing endocarditis on the supravalvular suture line, at least in the early postoperative period. Antibiotic prophylaxis is not required for cardiac biopsy or other invasive procedures performed by sterile technique. Table 3 outlines the current American Heart Association (AHA) recommendations for antibiotic prophylaxis. The only other currently used routine prophylactic regimen is sulfa/trimethoprim (Bactrim DS, two tablets daily, 3 days/week) as a highly effective measure to prevent infection with *Pneumocystis carinii*.

From: Smith JA, McCarthy PM, Sarris GE, Stinson EB, Reitz BA (eds.): The Stanford Manual of Cardiopulmonary Transplantation. Futura Publishing Co., Inc., Armonk, NY, 1996.

Table 1
Most Frequent Causes of Infections After Cardiac Transplantation in the
Stanford Series (1968 to 1994)

Type of Infection	Percentage
Bacterial	(43% of total)
Coliforms and Gram negatives	66
Staphylococcus	17
Legionella	6
Streptococcus	8
Listeria	3
Viral (Excluding *Herpes Simplex* virus and Human papilloma)	(37% of total)
Cytomegalovirus	48
Herpes zoster	43
Hepatitis B	6
Other	3
Fungal	(13% of total)
Aspergillus	54
Candida	24
Miscellaneous	22
Protozoan	(5% of total)
Pneumocystis	82
Toxoplasmosis	18
Nocardia	(2% of total)

Table 2
Total Bacterial Infections in Cardiac Transplant Recipients in the
Stanford Series (1968 to 1994)

Infection	Percentage	Infection	Percentage
E. coli	18.3	Proteus	1.9
Staphylococcus	14.3	Clostridium	1.7
Pseudomonas	11.0	Pneumococcus	1.6
Enterococci	7.5	Citrobacter	1.4
Streptococcus	6.9	Hemophilus	1.1
Serratia	6.3	Acinetobacter	<1.0
Klebsiella	5.8	Mycobacterium TB	<1.0
Enterobacter	5.7	Cat Scratch	<1.0
Anerobes	5.0	Mycoplasma	<1.0
Legionella	4.8	Atypical mycobacteria	<1.0
Listeria	2.5	Salmonella	<1.0

Table 3
Guidelines for Antibiotic Prophylaxis of Endocarditis

Dental and Upper Respiratory Procedures

Oral	Amoxicillin	3 gm 1 hour before procedure;
	or	then 1.5 gm 6 hours after initial dose
	Erythromycin	1 gm 2 hours before procedure;
		then 500 mg 6 hours after initial dose
Parenteral	Ampicillin	2 gm IV or IM 30 minutes before procedure
	and	and
	Gentamicin	1.5 mg/kg (not > 80 mg) 30 minutes before precedure; may repeat both once 8 hours after initial dose.

Gastrointestinal and Genitourinary Procedures

Oral	Amoxicillin	3 gm 1 hour before procedure; then 1.5 gm 6 hours after initial dose
Parenteral	Ampicillin	2 gm IV or IM 30 minues before procedure
	and	and
	Gentamicin	1.5 mg/kg (not > 80 mg) 30 minutes before procedure; may repeat both once 8 hours after initial dose.
	or	
	Vancomycin	1 gm IV over 1 hour, commencing 1 hour before procedure
	and	and
	Gentamicin	1.5 mg/kg (not > 80 mg) 1 hour before procedure; may repeat once 8 hours after initial dose.

Reproduced with permission from Dajani AS, Bisno AL, Chung KJ et al. Prevention of Bacterial Endocarditis. Recommendations by the American Heart Association. JAMA 1990;264: 2919–2922.

Workup of a Fever—General Aspects

History

The purpose of the history is to elicit symptoms that may localize the source of infection. A thorough history, physical exam, and basic laboratory studies (chest X-ray, urinalysis, hepatic and renal panels) will identify a site of infection in most cases and thus avoid extensive, random testing.

The following symptom complexes should be routinely queried:

Breathlessness, cough, sputum production, chest pain suggesting chest infection

Headache, photophobia, altered level of consciousness, concentration
   or personality change suggesting meningitis
Localized neurological signs indicating possible brain abscess
Dysuria and frequency suggesting urinary infection
Abdominal pain, jaundice, and change in bowel habits

A drug history should note any recent changes in the patient's drug regimen, possible drug interactions, and any interruption of prophylaxis because of pneumocystis or endocarditis. The patient's serologic status with regard to previous infection (cytomegalovirus [CMV], toxoplasma) should also be noted. The presence of any indwelling intravascular device or recent surgical wound should automatically lead to consideration of these as possible sources of infection. Patients should be instructed to report promptly any persistent fever > 38°C.

Cardiac rejection coexistent with infection should be considered and excluded early, particularly when CMV is found to be the causative organism (because of a strong association between active CMV infection and the presence of cardiac rejection). Rejection alone is not usually associated with a significant fever.

Physical Examination

Examination should be directed toward evidence of specific infection and should include the body systems and considerations as outlined in Table 4.

Table 4
Physical Examination for Evidence of Infection

Body Systems	Considerations
General	Temperature, heart rate, blood pressure, general appearance e.g., well-looking/toxic/septic/dyspneic
CVS	Heart sounds (murmurs), peripheral signs of shortness of breath on exertion
Resp	Respiratory rate, cyanosis, rales/creps/wheezes
GI	Abdominal or flank tenderness, hepatosplenomegaly, abdominal mass, rectal exam (guaiac testing of stools)
CNS	Meningismus, full neurological examination for localizing signs
Hematol	Lymphadenopathy
Head	Examination of oral cavity for ulceration, petechiae, etc.; tympanic membranes, facial sinus tenderness
Skin	Rash, ulcers, petechiae, blisters
Gen/Urinary	Discharge, ulceration, bleeding
Wounds if present	Signs of infection

Laboratory Investigations

Table 5 outlines the laboratory tests and procedures to be performed. All or some of them should be used as needed. Diagnostic methods and serologic tests may vary from institution to institution. Microbiological methods should be checked with the appropriate department. If chest X-rays are done, they should be compared with previous X-rays if infiltrates are subtle. Since the lung is the most common site of infections in cardiac transplant recipients, an aggressive approach to diagnosis and the availability of a skilled bronchoscopist are most important in caring for these patients.

Bacterial Infections

In general, bacterial infections in cardiac transplant recipients should be treated as they are in nontransplant patients. Early diagnosis is even more important in immunosuppressed patients, and empiric treatment for the most likely pathogen should be started as soon as all microbiological specimens have been obtained. Generally, we prefer double coverage with bactericidal antibiotics and continue treatment for several days longer than a standard course. The frequency of specific bacterial infections in the Stanford series in recipients treated with cyclosporine is presented in Table 2. The list contains many "ordinary" pathogens, but also a high incidence of "opportunistic" bacteria, several of which deserve individual comment below.

Table 5
Laboratory Investigations for Evidence of Infection

Areas	Tests or Procedures
Radiographic	Chest x-ray
	Bone x-ray
Cultures	Blood
	Urine
	Sputum
	Wound
	CMV
	CSF
Serology	Viral
	Other
Other Procedures	Abdominal CT Scan
	Bronchoscopy
	Endoscopy

Legionella

Infections due to Legionella species (fastidious Gram-negative bacteria found in soil, drinking water, and air conditioning units) are not uncommon and are often hospital acquired. In the past, pulmonary infections were the most common, but, recently, surgical wound infections and endocarditis have been reported.

Diagnosis

Transbronchial biopsy and bronchoalveolar lavage are required to identify the organism in pulmonary infections. A four-fold rise in serum direct fluorescent antibody (DFA) titer on paired sera may confirm the diagnosis. Specific media must be used for growth; therefore, the infection must be specifically sought. Culture takes 3–5 days.

Treatment

Erythromycin 500 mg-1 gm qid intravenously (IV) or orally for 14 days. Because erythromycin blocks hepatic metabolism of cyclosporine, thus resulting in markedly increased cyclosporine levels, the cyclosporine dose must be reduced when erythromycin is used. Cutting the cyclosporine dose in half and following drug levels carefully will, in most cases, prevent undue fluctuations in cyclosporine levels. Tetracycline is the second line agent. However, the soundest approach to hospital-acquired legionellosis, is to treat the institutional portable water system (e.g., hyperchlorination). We have also used the use of prophylactic perioperative use of erythromycin (500 mg IV preoperatively every 6 hours for a total of 48 hours). These measures have resulted in elimination of infection with Legionella at Stanford.

Listeria

Listeria monocytogenes, a Gram-positive organism, almost invariably causes meningeal infection, but it can also occasionally cause septicemia and endocarditis. Although the mode of transmission is obscure, it may involve the oral route from infected cheese products in some cases. Presenting symptoms may be extremely subtle but are usually those of any bacterial meningitis, including headaches, fever, nausea and vomiting, personality change, or difficulty in concentrating. Rarely, intracerebral abscess formation occurs.

Diagnosis

The diagnosis is based on identifying the organism on gram stain and culture of cerebrospinal fluid (CSF). A computerized tomographic (CT) brain scan should be pursued first to exclude a space-occupying lesion that could increase the risk of peduncular coning with lumbar puncture. Blood cultures, if positive, may be confirmatory, but serological tests are unreliable.

Treatment

For infections of the central nervous system with Listeria penicillin G (400,000 units/kg per day IV in six divided doses) or ampicillin (200–300 mg/kg per day IV in six divided doses) should be given. If the patient is allergic to penicillin, tetracycline is the next drug of choice at a recommended dose of 15 mg/kg per day IV in four divided doses.

Viral Infections

Herpes Simplex

Herpes simplex (HSV) is the most common viral infection after transplant surgery. It most frequently causes cold sores or oral ulcerations (HSV I), genital ulcerations (HSV II), and, rarely, esophageal and gastric ulceration (HSV I), which may lead to severe gastrointestinal hemorrhage.

Excluding HSV and human papilloma viral infections, which are extremely common, 62% of viral infections are due to CMV, 30% are due to Herpes zoster, 6% due to hepatitis B, and 3% to other agents including Influenza A, Epstein-Barr virus (EBV), and human T-cell Leukemia virus.

Diagnosis

A clinical diagnosis of mucocutaneous disease is enough to justify empiric treatment. Gastrointestinal disease, on the other hand, is not clinically distinguishable from other infectious causes of ulceration and requires endoscopy for culture specimens and histologic confirmation.

Treatment

Oral acyclovir (200 mg five times a day for 5 days) is recommended for mucocutaneous herpes. IV acyclovir is generally used for gastrointestinal disease, and the duration of therapy is determined by endoscopic proof of healing of the ulceration. In patients with normal renal function, the IV dosage is 5 mg/kg infused over 1 hour every 8 hours for 7 days. If there is significant renal impairment, the dosing interval must be adjusted as follows:

Creatinine Clearance (mls/min)	Dose (mg/kg)	Dose Interval (hours)
>50	5	8
25–50	5	12
10–25	5	24
0–10	2.5	24

Side effects include phlebitis if concentrated IV solutions are used, renal failure (precipitation of acyclovir crystals in the renal tubules), and, rarely, encephalopathic changes.

Recurrences of mucocutaneous lesions may be controlled by acyclovir (200 mg daily) in some patients or by patient-instituted therapy at the first sign of a new lesion. Chronic acyclovir prophylaxis for gastrointestinal disease has not proved to be effective, but it may be reasonable in selected patients.

Cytomegalovirus

CMV, a member of the herpes group of DNA viruses, is an endemic organism worldwide. It is a major cause of morbidity and mortality after cardiac transplantation. The risk of this and other herpes group viral infection is higher with immunosuppression therapy directed at cellular immune function (cyclosporine, ATG, OKT3), and the risk increases in older patients. The chance of developing CMV infection is related to several factors. Higher overall doses of immunosuppression (particularly antithymocyte globulin) increase the prevalence of CMV disease and the duration of viral shedding. Virus may be shed in urine, nasal and throat washings, and bronchoalveolar lavage fluid in many cardiac recipients who are seropositive preoperatively.

Transmission

CMV infection may result from a primary infection in a seronegative individual, reactivation in a previously infected individual, or reinfection with a new strain. Primary infections are more often clinically severe and life threatening and occur in the earlier posttransplant period on average than do cases of reactivation CMV.

Primary Infection. Primary infection occurs in a previously uninfected (seronegative) host. Sources include: 1. donor organ mismatch in which a seronegative recipient receives the heart of a seropositive donor; 2. blood transfusion in which CMV seropositive blood or blood products are given to a seronegative recipient (this can largely be avoided if only CMV-negative blood products are used for seronegative recipients); and 3. more usual sources, such as from close, prolonged contact with an infected individual or a CMV excreter. Seroconversion may occur quite late, or *not at all,* in primary disease.

Reactivation. Often CMV infection is a reactivation of a prior/latent infection in a seropositive individual after the immunosuppression or augmented immunosuppression has been started for rejection. In these cases, the clinical illness is usually, although not necessarily, mild.

Reinfection. Uncommonly, a primary infection with a different CMV strain may occur in a previously seropositive recipient. The resulting clinical illness is generally milder than that seen with a primary infection.

Symptoms

Symptoms and signs of CMV infection in immunosuppressed patients include fever, headache, arthralgias, abdominal pain (due to hepatitis or gastritis), diarrhea, or rash. Organ involvement can include pneumonitis, myocarditis, pericarditis, hepatitis, gastritis, colitis, chorioretinitis, leukopenia and anemia, and splenomegaly. Serious and life threatening manifestations such as pneumonitis, myocarditis, hepatitis, chorioretinitis, and gastritis are more common in the immunosuppressed host, whereas in non-immunosuppressed hosts CMV infections are usually subclinical.

Sequelae

Leukopenia, caused by viral bone marrow suppression, often accompanies CMV infection. It is, in fact, one of the earliest abnormalities detectable and often precedes the development of symptoms. The tendency to leukopenia is most marked in patients receiving azathioprine and, once profound, it may persist for up to 2 months despite early discontinuation of azathioprine.

Concomitant Infection

More than 50% of cardiac transplant recipients who develop CMV infection will suffer a concomitant bacterial, protozoan, or other viral infection.

Rejection

The incidence of cardiac rejection is also increased in the presence of CMV infection. It is not always clear whether rejection is caused by CMV infection or if the tendency to reject, with necessary augmentation of immunosuppression, predisposes to the infection.

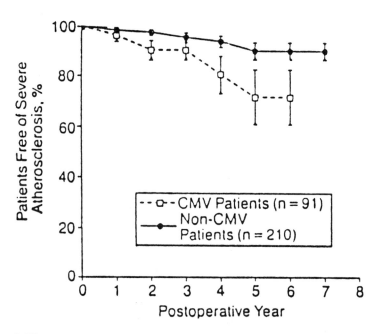

Figure 1. The actuarial rate of development of angiographically severe obstruction (> 70% luminal narrowing) in a major coronary artery was significantly greater in the cytomegalovirus (CMV) patients ($P < .05$). Development of coronary artery disease in CMV-positive patients. (Reproduced with permission from Grattan M, et al. JAMA 1989;261:3561–3566.)

Coronary Artery Disease

Patients with CMV infection after transplantation (whether symptomatic or not) are more likely to develop the late complication of graft coronary artery disease and to die as a result (Figure 1). This complication may be due to the association of CMV with increased cardiac rejection, to the predilection of CMV for endothelial cells with stimulation of intimal hyperplasia, or to other, as yet poorly understood, immunologic mechanisms.

Diagnosis

Many transplant centers rely on a latex fixation assay for total CMV antibody (IgG and IgM), which is reported as a titer (positive > 1/8). Enzyme-linked immunoadsorbent assay IgM-specific testing confirms the evidence of recent infection. Parallel testing of serial specimens is important to validate a suspected seroconversion or significant rise in titer.

Cultures. CMV may be cultured directly from pulmonary tissue, nasopharyngeal washings, throat, urine, or buffy coat preparations. CMV commonly takes 4–6 weeks to be grown in ordinary viral culture media. A newer, rapid method for culture is the shell vial culture in which the specimen is grown on tissue culture monolayer and stained with a monoclonal antibody against "early" CMV antigen. Results can be read at 24 and 48 hours. This rapid culture method cannot be used for any specimens containing serum and is thus not useful for buffy coat culture.

Tissues. Tissue biopsy is often the most rapid method for diagnosing CMV infection. Characteristic nucleolar CMV inclusion bodies may be detected in biopsy specimens of myocardium, GI tract, liver, or other tissue. Viral DNA hybridization techniques and viral cultures from such tissue may assist the diagnosis, but in situ hybridization has not proven to be more sensitive than routine histology.

Prevalence

Between 56%–100% of recipients are seropositive for CMV before transplantation (depending on age), and 40% of donors are positive. Around 10% of seropositive recipients develop clinical reactivation CMV, and it is higher for those who receive heavier immunosuppression because a seronegative recipient has a 30% chance of receiving the heart from a positive donor, this high risk situation results in a primary CMV infection in 70%–80% of seronegative recipients.

Treatment

DHPG (2-hydroxy-1-hydroxy methyl 1-ethoxymethyl guanine, ganciclovir; Syntex Laboratories, Palo Alto, CA, USA) is an antiviral agent that competitively inhibits virus-specific DNA polymerase. At present, its use is approved for life-threatening and sight-threatening CMV infections. Dosage is 5 mg/kg every 12 hours IV for 14 days. Its most serious and common side effect is leukopenia. The dosage should be reduced by 50%. If leukopenia is mild, and if the white cell count falls below 5,000/mm^3, it should be discontinued. Some patients (particularly those with gastritis or retinitis) require maintenance DHPG (5 mg/kg per day 3 days/week) for extended periods to control disease. Since DHPG is excreted mainly by the kidneys, the dose must be reduced in renally impaired patients, according to the following guidelines:

Creatinine Clearance (mLs/min)	DHPG Dose (IV, q 12 hours)
<25	1.25 mg/kg
25–49	2.5 mg/kg
50–80	2.5 mg/kg
>80	5.0 mg/kg

The use of acyclovir may be considered where leukopenia precludes use of DHPG, although its effectiveness in CMV infections has not been established. Importantly, azathioprine often must be reduced or discontinued when CMV infection is associated with leukopenia.

Leukopenia from viral infection and/or treatment with DHPG and azathioprine is not uncommon. A new drug, filgrastin, was recently released by the US Food and Drug Administration as the first of a pioneering class of drugs. The drug is a granulocyte colony stimulating factor that is indicated for severe leukopenia (absolute neutrophil count <500/mm^3) to treat episodes of infection or to prevent infection. Although it has primarily been used for patients receiving chemotherapy, it may also be useful for transplant patients.

Prophylaxis

Cytomegalovirus Hyperimmune Globulin.   Some transplant centers have reported that the severity of primary CMV infections is reduced in seroneg-

ative recipients treated with varying regimens of CMV hyperimmune globulin in the early postoperative period. Its role is not yet established, however disadvantages include the high cost and a small risk of transmission of
HIV or hepatitis B viruses.

DHPG.   In a study at Stanford (in collaboration with the Utah Cardiac
Transplant Program) the frequency and severity of CMV infection were reduced when DHPG was used daily for the first 14 postoperative days. This
randomized, double-blind, placebo-controlled study of prophylactic DHPG
after heart transplantation involved 148 adult patients who were seropositive at the time of transplantation or received a graft from a seropositive
donor (or both). Treatment consisted of DHPG 5 mg/kg IV every 12 hours
(adjusted downward for impaired creatinine clearance) or placebo for 14
days beginning on the first postoperative day, followed by DHPG 6 mg/kg
IV or placebo five times/week for 2 more weeks. The total incidence of
CMV disease was highly significantly reduced in DHPG-treated recipients.
It included proven, specific organ involvement as well as CMV "syndrome"
(positive cultures plus two of the following: fever, hepatic dysfunction,
leukopenia/thrombocytopenia). CMV excretion was significantly reduced
at 2, 4, and 8 weeks postoperatively in the drug treatment group. No significant difference was found in the incidence of adverse events in the two
groups. This study confirmed an important beneficial effect of prophylactic DHPG treatment after heart transplantation in seropositive recipients,
according to the drug schedule used in the study. Whether a more abbre-
viated course would be as efficacious has not been determined. In seronegative patients, it was felt that more prolonged prophylaxis would potentially
be of benefit. Therefore, for these patients, an additional 2 weeks of DHPG
prophylaxis (6 mg/kg IV, five times/week) is used.

Donors Matching to Recipients.   In theory, it would be preferable to give
only CMV-seronegative donor hearts to CMV-negative recipients. Although
such a strict matching scheme is often not logistically possible, blood products should at least be screened, and only CMV-negative transfusions of
blood and platelets should be used in CMV-negative recipients.

Herpes Zoster

Recrudescence of *Varicella zoster* (chicken pox) virus ("shingles") often
occurs in transplant recipient. It usually presents as a painful vesicular rash

in a unilateral dermatomal distribution, but tingling or pain in one or more dermatomes may precede the rash by several days. Treatment with acyclovir (200 mg po five times/day) may shorten the duration of rash. The development of postherpetic neuralgia is the most serious sequela of this infection, and it can be quite difficult to manage. Although carbamazepine is used to treat this condition with some success, carbamazepine induces the hepatic enzyme system that metabolizes cyclosporine and predictably leads to an increase in the cyclosporine requirement.

Epstein-Barr Virus

Clinical Considerations

EBV is endemic in the American population. Infection in the immunocompetent individual is usually subclinical, but it can present as an acute syndrome known as infectious mononucleosis. The true incidence of EBV infection after transplantation is not known, as evidence is not as commonly sought as that for other viruses mentioned in this section. This herpes family virus can be transmitted by the oropharyngeal route or by transfusion, and clinical infection may include headache, malaise, myalgia, fatigue, sore throat, palatal petechiae, lymphadenopathy, splenomegaly, hepatitis, and aseptic meningitis. It can also cause a chronic relapsing fever and a malaise syndrome, and may occur concomitantly with CMV infection. Long-term EBV infection appears to be associated with the development of lymphoma (see Chapter 8).

Diagnosis

Diagnosis is made primarily from serological tests, including EBV capsid antigen, EBV early antigen, and EBV specific IgM. The virus cannot be grown in culture, and no specific appearance is seen on biopsy specimens, although DNA probes can detect viral genomes in infected cells.

Treatment

Treatment is symptomatic. No specific antiviral agents have proven useful, although the empiric use of acyclovir in EBV-related lymphoma is currently advocated.

Human Papilloma Virus

Human papilloma virus (HPV) infection is common after transplantation. Many patients develop cutaneous warts that require control with diathermy, cautery, or astringent treatment. Warts tend to be multiple, recurrent, and resistant to treatment. HPV genital infection is a major concern in immunosuppressed women. Carriage of HPV (particularly oncogenic strains whether symptomatic or not is more frequent in immunosuppressed women. Female transplant recipients over 15 years of age should have Papanicolaou smear examination initially and at 6-month intervals to provide early detection of HPV-related cervical dysplasia and carcinoma.

Fungal Infections

The most common fungal infections that occur after cardiac transplantation are due to Aspergillus species, which account for 54% of all such infections. Candida species account for 30%, and 16% of fungal infections are due to miscellaneous organisms, including *Coccidioides immitis, Cryptococcus neoformans, Histoplasma capsulatum,* agents of mucormycosis (including Rhizopus and Mucor), and rarely, mycetomas due to fungi such as *Allescheria boydii.*

Aspergillus

Clinical Considerations

Infections with Aspergillus species most commonly involve the lung and often present as an asymptomatic nodule on the chest X-ray. Disseminated infection may involve the thoracic spine, sinuses, pleura, liver, spleen, joints, brain, thyroid, adrenal gland, and the transplanted heart. Symptoms depend on the site of infection, but they generally include fever and malaise. Of 30 cases of aspergillosis in the Stanford experience, 19 presented in lung, 9 were disseminated, 1 occurred in bone, and 1 patient had retinal disease. Disseminated aspergillus infections are associated with a very high death rate, despite adequate treatment with amphotericin, and a delay in making the diagnosis can contribute to higher death rates. For this reason, a very aggressive approach to the diagnosis of suspicious lesions is recommended.

Diagnosis

Diagnosis can be made by bone biopsy, fine needle pulmonary aspiration, or open lung biopsy. Bone biopsy specimens treated with potassium hydroxide provide direct demonstration of characteristic branching septate hyphae with histologic evidence of invasion. Culture of the fungus is confirmatory. Tests for the presence of antibody or antigen are not widely available nor generally accepted as useful.

Treatment

Depending upon the site of infection, surgical debridement of an affected area (especially bone) may be helpful in management. Amphotericin is the only antifungal antibiotic shown to be effective in controlling infection, and it can only be administered IV. Therapy is generally long-term, facilitated by establishing a semipermanent central venous access site. Before amphotericin administration patients are usually premedicated with hydrocortisone, aspirin, acetaminophen, antihistamine, and antiemetics because of the high incidence of systemic reactions to amphotericin. An initial test dose of 1 mg should be given over 60–120 minutes and heparin 1,000 units added to each infusion to reduce thrombophlebitis. If this test dose is well tolerated, the dosage can be titrated upward until 0.6 mg/kg per day is reached. After 1–2 weeks, if there is evidence of response, the dosage can be cut back to 0.6 mg/kg per day three times/week. Since the drug is highly nephrotoxic, its administration must be titrated according to the patient's renal function, and the dosage reduced or withheld if the serum creatinine exceeds 3 mg/dL. Unlike other antibiotics, the goal with amphotericin is generally a total cumulative dose of 2–3 gm rather than a total duration of therapy. The treatment period is often prolonged by nephrotoxicity that necessitates a slower rate of administration.

The new oral (triazol) antifungal agent itraconazole (recently FDA approved), has proved effective in treating several fungal infections, including those due to Aspergillus species, Candida, Cryptococcus, dermatophytes, and Coccidioides. It is less toxic than amphotericin, but interferes with the hepatic metabolism and possibly with the distribution of cyclosporine. The cyclosporine dosage must be approximately halved when itraconazole is started, in order to avoid toxic cyclosporine levels. Cyclosporine levels and renal function must be carefully monitored throughout administration. The drug is started at 400 mg bid for 5 days, then reduced to a maintenance of 200 mg bid (maximum 200 mg tid). Although side effects are uncommon, they may include headache, mild gastrointestinal symptoms, rash, urinary frequency, impotence, and gynecomastia. Associated laboratory abnormalities have included increased hepatic transaminase levels and occasionally hypokalemia. No life-threatening reactions have been reported.

Candida

Clinical Considerations

Manifestations of Candida infection after transplantation can include mucocutaneous infection, esophagitis, or sepsis due to intravascular or disseminated disease. Less commonly, hematogenous spread may occur to the lungs, skin, meninges, joints, bones, or even brain. Once disseminated, candidiasis tends to be rapidly fatal.

Diagnosis

Diagnosis requires that characteristic pseudohyphae be identified on wet smear of fluid or tissue, evidence of invasion on histologic sections, or culture from appropriate body fluids.

Prophylaxis

Nystatin is recommended qid in the early posttransplant period to prevent mucocutaneous infection either in a liquid suspension for "swish and swallow" or as throat lozenges.

Treatment

Ketaconazole (200 mg/day) is generally used to treat mucocutaneous Candida infections. Because side effects include hepatic toxicity, the patient's liver function should be monitored and the drug discontinued if elevations occur and persist. The dose should be given 2 hours before any antacids or H_2 blockers. Since ketaconazole inhibits liver metabolism of cyclosporine, the cyclosporine dosage must be decreased accordingly. In more widespread disease, amphotericin should be used as described for infections with Aspergillus. The use of itraconazole for disseminated candidal disease remains experimental.

Cryptococcus

Clinical Considerations

Cryptococcus neoformans, a yeast-like fungus, is an opportunistic pathogen that may be inhaled from dried pigeon droppings. Although it usually causes infection without an obvious exposure history, infection is thought to start in the lungs with granuloma and to spread later to the brain, skin, or bone. Clinically, headache, nausea, gait disturbances, meningismus, cranial nerve palsies, pulmonary infiltrates or effusions, skin papules, or osteolytic bone lesions may occur.

Diagnosis

Encapsulated yeast may be identified on India ink smear of CSF, and additionally, cryptococcal capsular antigen may be positive in CSF. Culture of CSF or other appropriate fluids or tissue may also confirm the diagnosis.

Treatment

Amphotericin is the first line agent (see section on Aspergillus).

The addition of flucytosine (5-FC) has proved synergistic in some cases and can reduce the dose of amphotericin needed for adequate therapy of cryptococcosis. Since 5-FC is excreted by the kidneys, its use in combination with cyclosporine and amphotericin is problematic, a problem made more complex by the fact that 5-FC and its metabolites are also toxic to the bone marrow. Most transplant recipients are also receiving azathioprine in doses previously titrated to marrow tolerance, so that careful monitoring of blood counts is essential, with titration of the dose of azathioprine when necessary.

Determining the minimal inhibitory concentration of the organism for amphotericin and itraconazole may facilitate a decision about whether to add 5-FC. CSF and serum cryptococcal antigen levels may be used to monitor the response to antimicrobial therapy.

Coccidioides

Clinical Considerations

Coccidioides immitis is a soil saprophyte common in certain geographically specific areas, and inhalation is generally thought to be the mode of transmission. Clinical symptoms include a mild flu-like illness, pneumonia, arthritis, conjunctivitis, chronic pulmonary granulomatous lesions, infiltrates, or effusions. Infection has been associated with *Erythema nodosum* or *multiforme* in immunosuppressed patients.

Diagnosis

Diagnosis can be made by examining tissue on fluid specimens. Serologic tests may be positive if the disease is widespread, although results tend to be negative with solitary lung lesions. Confirmation by culture from appropriate specimens is needed for a definitive diagnosis.

Treatment

Amphotericin should be used for treatment, as well as surgical debridement when feasible. Itraconazole is being investigated for treatment of coccidioidal infections and may prove to be a useful alternative to amphotericin.

Protozoan Infections

Of protozoan infections in the Stanford experience, 89% were due to Pneumocystitis and the remaining 11% were due to Toxoplasma.

Pneumocystis

Pulmonary infection with the protozoan pathogen *Pneumocystis carinii* has been less common since effective prophylaxis with sulfa/trimethoprim was introduced. Now, in fact, this infection rarely occurs except when prophylaxis has been interrupted or not used. Site of infection is usually restricted to the lungs. The infection may occur any time from 6 weeks after transplantation, often coincident with another opportunistic infection. This organism is a common respiratory tract commensal in a majority of the normal population.

Symptoms

Symptoms can include breathlessness, dry cough, fever, fatigue, and malaise. On examination cyanosis and progressive hypoxemia, sometimes to a degree requiring ventilatory support, can occur. Respiratory symptoms are classically more marked than suggested by chest X-ray changes in the early stages, and signs are often minimal at first. After some days, a characteristic diffuse reticular bilateral infiltrate can generally be seen on the chest X-ray, although radiographic findings vary greatly.

Diagnosis

The diagnosis can be suspected on the basis of typical symptoms associated with characteristic chest X-ray changes and hypoxemia. However, it must be confirmed by demonstration of the organism in appropriate tissue specimens, usually bronchoalveolar lavage fluid, using Gomori methenamine silver stain to identify the cyst form of the organism and sometimes Giemsa stain to identify the trophozoite form.

Prophylaxis

Pneumocystis infections can largely be prevented after transplantation by use of sulfa/trimethoprim tablets bid 3 days/week. In patients who cannot tolerate sulfa/trimethoprim because of allergy or leukopenia, pentamidine 300 mg once monthly administered as a nebulized solution, by inhalation is an alternative form of prophylaxis. However, pentamidine is considered a less effective prophylactic regimen, than sulfa/trimethoprim. Several reports have described disseminated nonpulmonary pneumocystis infection in acquired immune deficiency syndrome patients who received pentamidine prophylaxis by inhalation.

Treatment

Pneumocystis infections should be treated with trimethoprim 20 mg/kg per day and sulfamethoxazole 100 mg/kg per day IV in four divided doses for 14 days. Oral therapy can be substituted in the latter part of the treatment course if the patient is clinically well. Side effects of sulfa therapy include skin rash and nausea. The drug is mildly toxic to the bone marrow, and leukopenia and thrombocytopenia, especially in patients taking azathioprine, may be seen. Treatment is usually successful if started early in the course of infection, but deaths have occurred, especially in cases of mixed infections.

For patients who cannot take sulfa/trimethoprim, pentamidine isethionate (4 mg/kg once daily IM or IV for 14 days) is the alternative choice. IV infusions should be given over 1 hour to limit the potential hypotensive reaction. Other side effects include leukopenia, thrombocytopenia, and hypoglycemia.

Toxoplasmosis

The protozoan organism *Toxoplasma gondii* is not a common cause of infection in cardiac transplant recipients, but it can present as a fulminating disseminated infection in seronegative individuals who become infected.

Clinical Considerations

Clinical manifestations can include fever, headache, polymyositis, pericarditis, encephalitis, rash, hepatosplenomegaly, lymphadenopathy, pneumonitis, hepatitis, chorioretinitis, and myocarditis. Asymptomatic seroconversions can occur. As with CMV, transmission to a previously uninfected (seronegative) transplant recipient may occur by means of: 1. direct primary infection (i.e., toxoplasmosis cysts in the donor heart implanted into recipient; 2. blood transfusion (uncommon); and 3. other sources (ingested pork or lamb, contact with cat feces). Reactivation is rare in seropositive patients.

Diagnosis

Depending on the suspected site of infection, serological tests and possibly some of the following should be performed: retinal examination; lymph node biopsy; myocardial biopsy; liver biopsy; and CT brain scan.

At Stanford, the Sabin-Feldman dye test is used for total IgG and IgM antitoxoplasma antibodies. An IgG titer of 1:16 is considered low positive. A double sandwich ELISA test for IgM is used to confirm the occurrence of recent infection. Testing of serial samples from the same individual in parallel is important to establish definite titer changes over time. Cysts or parasites may be identified in tissue specimens (including graft biopsies) stained with either hematoxylin eosin or with Giemsa stain.

Prevalence

Around 30% of recipients and 40% of donors are seropositive preoperatively. Seropositivity in the recipient appears to confer immunity regardless of the donor's serologic status. Mismatch results, however (i.e., seropositive donor into seronegative recipient), results in clinical disease in 10%–60% of cases, depending on levels of immunosuppression. This risk is undoubtedly highest when the donor is IgM positive.

Treatment

The treatment of choice is combined pyrimethamine and sulfonamides (sulfadiazine or trisulfapyrimidines). A loading dose of pyrimethamine 50–100 mg orally on day 1 and then 25-mg daily thereafter is used. Sulfadiazine or trisulfapyrimidines at a loading dose of 4 gm, followed by 1 gm four times/day thereafter is advised. If started early in the disease, treatment is usually successful, but it should be continued for 3–6 months. Side effects of pyrimethamine include marrow suppression. The administration of folinic acid once or twice a week to reduce marrow toxicity is controversial. Spiramycin has been used successfully in Europe. Prophylaxis with pyrimethamine for mismatched recipients may be effective in preventing clinical disease, but this treatment remains unproved.

Actinomycetes

Clinical Considerations

Infection with Nocardia species (*N. asteroides, brasiliensis, caviae*) is not uncommon in cardiac transplant recipients. These aerobic actinomycetes are classified as true bacteria although they tend to filamentous growth with true branching. They are ubiquitous soil saprophytes that most commonly infect humans via the respiratory tract, they produce suppurative lesions characterized by acute necrosis and abscess formation. Extension to the pleura or chest wall often produces empyema, subcutaneous abscess, or osteomyelitis, and hematogenous spread can lead to widely disseminated infection with abscess formation in the brain or other viscera, sometimes in the absence of obvious pulmonary infection. Although the disease is rarely fulminant, it can pursue an extremely chronic, persistent course. True cure of extrapulmonary disease in the immunosuppressed host is rare.

Diagnosis

Serologic testing for Nocardia is not available, but it is usually not difficult to identify the characteristic weakly Gram-positive, weakly acid fast, branching hyphae in sputum, bronchoalveolar lavage, or appropriate tissue specimens. The organism grows on standard bacterial culture medium but can take up to 10 days to grow. The microbiology laboratory should be instructed to "hold for nocardia" any specimen suspected to contain this organism (since specimens are often discarded after 7 days).

Treatment

Therapy for Nocardia infection should include surgical drainage of any suppurative, closed space infection whenever feasible. In many cases surgical therapy involves multiple drainage procedures, drainage tubes, and occasionally limb amputation. Sulfa treatment is the mainstay of chemotherapy, and sulfadiazine in a dose of 4–6 gm/day or more in divided doses is recommended. However, marrow toxicity (especially in patients already taking azathioprine) may preclude use of such high doses. Second-line drugs include minocycline, ampicillin, and erythromycin. In vitro sensitivity can be pursued in some reference labs and may provide guidance in choice of a second-line drug when this is necessary. Duration of required therapy is uncertain. For isolated pulmonary lesions that resolve promptly, 6 months of drug therapy is generally considered adequate; however, for more widespread infection, lifetime therapy is usually necessary.

Selected References

1. Denning D, Tucker R, Hansen L, et al. Treatment of invasive aspergillosis with itraconazole. Am J Med 1989;86:791–800.
2. Gabrilove JL, Jakubowski A, Scher H, et al. Effectiveness of granulocyte colony stimulating factor on neutropenia and associated morbidity due to chemotherapy for transitional cell carcinoma of the urothelium. N Engl J Med 1988;318: 1414–1422.
3. Grattan M, Moreno-Cabral C, Starnes V, et al. CMV is associated with cardiac allograft rejection and atherosclerosis. JAMA 1989;261:3561–3566.
4. Hakim M, Esmore D, Wallwork J, et al. Toxoplasmosis in cardiac transplantation. Br Med J 1986;292:1108.
5. Icenogle T, Peterson E, Ray G, et al. DHPG effectively treats cytomegalovirus infection in heart and heart-lung transplant patients: A preliminary report. J Heart Transplant 1987;5:390.
6. Jamieson S, Oyer P, Reitz B. Cardiac transplantation at Stanford. J Heart Transplant 1981;1:86–91.
7. Johnson A, Gu Q, Roberts H. Antibody patterns in the serological diagnosis of acute lymphadenopathic toxoplasmosis. Aust N Z J Med 1987;17:430–434.
8. Keating MR, Wilhelm MP, Walker RC. Strategies for prevention of infection after cardiac transplantation. Mayo Clin Proc 1992;67:676–684.

9. Kramer M, Marshall S, Denning D, et al. Cyclosporine and itraconazole interaction in heart and lung transplant recipients. Ann Intern Med 1990;113:327–329.

10. Luft B, Billingham M, Remington J. Endomycardial biopsy in the diagnosis of toxoplasmic myocarditis. Transplant Proc 1986;18:1871–1873.

11. Merigan TC, Renlund DG, Keay S, et al. A controlled trial of ganciclovir to prevent cytomegalovirus disease after heart transplantation. N Engl J Med 1992; 326:1182–1186.

12. McGregor C, Fleck D, Nagington J, et al. Disseminated toxoplasmosis in cardiac transplantation. J Clin Pathol 1984;37:74–77.

13. Onorato I, Morens D, Martone W, et al. Epidemiology of cytomegaloviral infections: Recommendatins for prevention and control. Rev Infect Dis 1985;4: 479–497.

14. Pollard R, Arvin A, Gamberg P, et al. Specific cell-mediated immunity and infections with herpes viruses in cardiac transplant recipients. Am J Med 1982;73: 679–687.

15. Preiksaitis J, Rorno S, Rasmussen L, et al. CMV infection in heart transplant recipients: Role of the donor heart and immunosuppressive therapy. J Infect Dis 1983;147:974–981.

16. Rand K, Pollard R, Merigan T. Increased pulmonary superinfections in cardiac transplant recipients undergoing primary CMV infection. N Engl J Med 1978; 298:951–953.

17. Schafers H, Milbradt H, Flik J, et al. Hyperimmune globulin for CMV prophylaxis following heart transplantation. Clin Transpl 1988;2:51–56.

18. Watson F, O'Connell J, Amber I, et al. Treatment of CMV pneumonia in heart transplant recipients with DHPG. J Heart Transplant 1987;5:390.

19. Wreghitt TG, Gray JJ, Balfour AH. Problems with serological diagnosis of toxoplasmosis gondii in heart transplant recipients. J Clin Pathol 1986;39:1135–1139.

20. Yee GC. GM-CSS G-CSF: Promising biotherapeutics for use in hematology and oncology. Hosp Formul 1990;25:943–948.

Chapter 8

Follow-Up, Late Problems, and Results of Cardiac Transplantation

Anne M. Keogh, M.B., B.S., M.D., FRACP,
Julian A. Smith, M.B., M.S., FRACS,
George E. Sarris, M.D., Sharon A. Hunt, M.D.,
Joan Miller, R.N.

Rejection and infectious complications are most frequent in the first 3 months posttransplant, and are often insidious in onset. Frequent monitoring during this period is critical to detect complications early enough to successfully treat them. Regular follow-up is thus scheduled. Unscheduled, immediate consultation for any new symptoms, no matter how subtle, is actively encouraged. In an uncomplicated patient, a routine monitoring schedule is usually followed (Table 1).

Initially, once weekly chest film, complete blood count, renal and hepatic function, electrolytes, cholesterol/triglycerides, and trough cyclosporine level are obtained, the results are checked and necessary drug adjustments are made. Electrocardiogram (ECG) is performed monthly.

Coronary angiography is performed yearly to detect coronary artery disease (CAD). If at 6-years posttransplant there is no evidence of CAD, this may be reduced to every 2 years in selected patients. When there is concern about the development of CAD, or the possibility of pre-existent CAD in the donor heart, unscheduled angiography may be performed at any time posttransplant. Intracoronary ultrasound (ICUS) has recently been performed in association with coronary angiography at Stanford. Echocardiography or MUGA scanning may be useful when there is concern about ventricular systolic function.

Causes of death posttransplant in the Stanford program are presented in Table 2.

From: Smith JA, McCarthy PM, Sarris GE, Stinson EB, Reitz BA (eds.): The Stanford Manual of Cardiopulmonary Transplantation. Futura Publishing Co., Inc., Armonk, NY, 1996.

151

Table 1
Routine Surveillance Schedule

Time Posttransplant	Scheduled Visits	Biopsies
Weeks 2–4	twice weekly	weekly
Weeks 5–12	weekly	biweekly
Month 3–6	monthly	monthly
Month 7 onward	every 6 weeks	every 3 months

Table 2
Causes of Death Following Cardiac Transplantation at Stanford

Cause	Percentage
Infection	35%
Rejection	17.2%
Graft Coronary Disease	17.2%
Nonlymphoid malignancy	5.5%
Nonspecific graft failure	4.7%
Pulmonary embolus	1.6%
Pulmonary hypertension	3.9%
Lymphoid malignancy	3.9%
Cerebrovascular disease	3.1%
Other	7.8%

Late Problems

Transplant Coronary Artery Disease

Graft coronary artery disease (TxCAD) leading to ischemia with consequent loss of ventricular function, myocardial infarction, or death remains the major factor limiting the longer term results of cardiac transplantation (Figure 1) and represents the major indication for retransplantation. It has been a documented problem in the pre- and post-cyclosporine eras of immunosuppression and occurs in as many as 42% of survivors by 5-years posttransplant. It has been documented to occur as early as 6 weeks following transplantation.

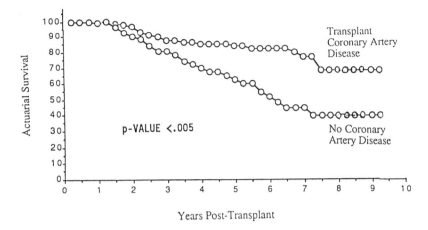

Figure 1. Actuarial survival after the development of transplant CAD. Survival is significantly reduced in those patients who develop CAD compared with those who do not.

Pathophysiology

The underlying cause or causes of the development of TxCAD in the cardiac allograft are not well understood, but seem to be quite different from those leading to the development of "ordinary" CAD. The disease is as common in those patients whose underlying heart disease was idiopathic cardiomyopathy as it is in those who previously had end-stage ischemic disease, and it is thus not easily related to the existence of the traditionally accepted risk factors for the development of CAD. Even the role of hyperlipidemia is controversial and not well shown. In a recent analysis of the long-term results of cardiac transplantations at Stanford in the cyclosporine era, older donor and recipient age emerged as independent risk factors for the development of TxCAD by multivariate analysis. Although a decline in incidence of TxCAD was shown, this could not be attributed to more potent immunosuppression with OKT3.

Nonetheless, an underlying immunologic phenomenon leading to initial injury of the coronary endothelium and gradually leading to TxCAD is the most attractive concept to many investigators. It is clear, however, that the occurrence of the usual biopsy diagnosed acute rejection episode correlates in only a general sort of way with the late occurrence of TxCAD. Recent observations of a high degree of correlation between evidence of postoperative cytomegalovirus (CMV) infection with the later development of

CAD may provide the first insights into the real mechanism of the disease, but this work is quite preliminary. The proposed mechanisms involve virally-mediated injury to the coronary endothelium and possible induction of humorally-mediated rejection, which may also damage coronary endothelium.

A better understanding of the pathophysiology of this important post-transplant complication may lead to the development of logical means of prevention in years to come.

Morphology

Cardiac allograft coronary disease differs angiographically in several major respects from that seen in "ordinary" CAD. While transplant patients occasionally do develop discrete proximal stenoses of major epicardial vessels, the most common form of coronary disease is that of diffuse, primarily distal vessel concentric and longitudinal narrowing leading to distal vessel loss or "pruning". Collateral vessel formation is quite unusual in TxCAD.

At a histologic level, this disease appears to consist primarily of diffuse myointimal hyperplasia in its early stages, and later progresses to include lipid infiltration and typical plaque formation. Calcification is a fairly late occurrence.

Clinical

The development of allograft CAD may be extremely rapid. Recent demonstration of normal coronary angiographic appearance in no way excludes the possibility of interval development of graft coronary disease, even over periods as short as several weeks. Clinical suspicion should lend to repeat angiography.

Because the transplanted heart is denervated, patients do not experience classical angina. In fact, some patients do report highly atypical neck and arm pain, but a high degree of suspicion is required to recognize this as a possible angina equivalent and to differentiate it from the more common musculoskeletal and sternum-related chest pains.

Clinical manifestations may include myocardial infarction (painless), with malaise, diaphoresis, nausea, relative hypotension or shock, arrhythmias, and cardiac failure. The differential diagnosis includes acute cardiac rejection, nonspecific graft failure, and humoral rejection. Development of new ECG changes in asymptomatic patients has led to the diagnosis in a number of patients.

Cardiac failure may develop more gradually when less critical coronary arterial obstruction occurs or small branches are lost and result in cumulative subclinical small infarcts that eventually exceed a clinical threshold.

Sudden death is not uncommon and presumably is related to arrhythmias.

Detection

Routine annual coronary angiography is recommended and is generally accepted as the only means of detecting early disease. Intimal hyperplasia may cause very smooth and diffuse luminal narrowing, and even severe disease can be missed by this method unless careful comparisons are made of serial angiograms to look for distal "pruning" and branch loss.

Stress exercise testing is generally not useful because of baseline resting ECG changes (IRBBB, RBBB, or rarely LBBB) present in most patients, and the role of thallium scanning is not well established (it appears to be relatively insensitive).

ICUS is a reliable method of serially studying the progression of Tx-CAD. Moderate or severe intimal hyperplasia can be identified with ICUS in patients with no angiographic evidence of TxCAD. Accurate quantitiative information on vessel wall morphology and lumen dimension may be obtained.

Results

At Stanford, 25% of survivors have developed angiographically detected TxCAD of some degree by 5-years posttransplant. Accelerated graft atherosclerosis is the leading indication for retransplantation. Once CAD has developed, expected survival falls significantly (Figure 1).

Treatment

Because of the diffuse nature of the process, saphenous vein coronary artery bypass grafting has not been attempted at Stanford. Percutaneous transluminal coronary angioplasty (PTCA) has been used with temporary success in several patients with localized proximal coronary artery stenosis, but is generally recognized to be a palliative measure at best.

Retransplantation remains the most effective therapy. The timing of this is controversial, but, in general, those who are suitable for retransplantation are listed as soon as multi-vessel disease not amenable to PTCA is recognized. Retransplantation for TxCAD has been performed success-fully in 37 patients to date, including 2 third transplants, but the incidence of recurrent CAD in the second graft is high (50% of those who survive the first year).

No medical treatment has thus far been shown to be beneficial. Aspirin should be continued and aggressive attempts made to control serum cho-lesterol levels. No data are available regarding the role of beta-blockers.

Prophylaxis

Prophylaxis of TxCAD has been attempted with various doses of as-pirin and dipyridamole in the past. To date, there is no evidence that dipyri-damole or aspirin are effective in preventing graft atherosclerosis, although a randomized trial has never been (and probably never will be) performed. Aspirin (in platelet inhibitory doses of 80 mg/day) is still continued in the expectation that it may be shown to be effective in lessening graft coronary disease, similar to its effect in retarding saphenous vein graft disease. When gastrointestinal side effects ensue, low-dose, enteric-coated aspirin should be tried. Use of dipyridamole has been gradually reduced because of its side effect profile (headache, flushing), expense and lack of definite benefit. The calcium channel blocker, diltiazem, has been studied in an ongoing randomized protocol and has been shown to be associated with significantly less progression of coronary disease in the intermediate term (2–3 years posttransplant). The late results are as yet unknown.

Clearly, the development of rationally directed modes of prophylaxis awaits further insight into the basic pathophysiology of the process.

Lymphomas and Other Malignancies

Lymphoma

General.   Lymphoproliferative malignancies are the most common non-cutaneous tumors developing after cardiac and other whole organ trans-plants and are probably related to overall level of immunosuppression. They have been more common since the use of cyclosporine. Epstein-Barr virus (EBV) particles have been identified in lymphoma specimens (partic-ularly via DNA hybridization techniques), and serological evidence of ac-tive infection is often found around the time of development of the lymphoproliferative complication. A possible causative role for this virus has thus been proposed. Lymphomas may occur within months of commencing immunosuppression and may be multi-focal as well as multi-clonal in origin.

To date, 13 lymphomas have been detected in cardiac transplant recipients at Stanford since the introduction of cyclosporine. Site of origin was lymph node in 4, lung in 4, subcutaneous nodule in 2, and gastrointestinal in 1. Two further cases were diagnosed only at autopsy (heart, kidney, and bowel).

As expected, symptoms depend on site of origin. Lymphomas posttransplant are often extranodal and not uncommonly occur in the central nervous system. Evidence of hepatosplenomegaly and lymphadenopathy should be sought at every review of transplant recipients. Occasionally, generalized lymphadenopathy and fever may comprise a syndrome difficult to distinguish from infectious mononucleosis.

Pathology.   Lymphoma may be of large, small, or mixed cell type, be monoclonal or polyclonal, and is often immunoblastic and poorly differentiated. Non-Hodgkin's lymphoma predominates. Immunoperoxidase staining for secretion of kappa and lambda light chains help to differentiate lymphoma clonality. Most transplant related lymphomas are of B cell origin. A minority originate from a T-cell lineage.

Diagnosis.   Tests required after the initial diagnosis of lymphoma depend on the site of involvement expected and follow the usual format for lymphoma staging. Biopsies of lymph nodes suspected to be involved, liver, and any pulmonary nodules are required along with abdominal and chest CT scans and routine bone marrow biopsy. Staging laparotomy is not usually pursued.

Treatment.   Lymphoma arising in the immunosuppressed patient does not, in the main, respond to usual treatment with radio- and chemotherapy. Rather, because of its relation to immunosuppression, minimization of immunosuppression (reduction/cessation of cyclosporine, reduction/cessation of azathioprine, and increase in prednisone) can lead to resolution of lymphoma deposits over a period of a few months. Failure to reduce immunosuppression invariably results in progression of lymphoma to death.

Depending on site of origin and its sequelae (e.g., localized lymphoma leading to GI perforation) surgical excision of the tumor may have a role. Because of the association with EBV, long-term oval acyclovir has been advocated, although its efficacy in this setting is not yet proven; however, we have used it routinely in both adults and children. These tumors seem generally to be radiosensitive and the role of localized adjunctive radiotherapy should not be underestimated. The potential adverse sequelae of decreasing immunosuppression in these patients is obvious; appropriately timed serial biopsies are, therefore, necessary.

Solid Malignancies

In general, the incidence of nonlymphoproliferative malignancies is not expected to be higher following solid organ transplantation. Skin malignancies, and carcinoma of the vulva and perineum appear to be the exception, and should be carefully sought, biopsied early, and treated aggressively.

To date, 14 patients have developed solid organ malignancy post-transplantation and one suffered recurrence of a previously treated bowel malignancy. Those 14 instances of malignancy arising de novo posttransplant included 5 lung carcinomas (4 adenocarcinomas and 1 squamous cell carcinoma [SCC]), 5 colon adenocarcinomas (2 with liver metastases), 1 hypernephroma, 1 prostatic adenocarcinoma, 1 cervical adenocarcinoma, and 1 hepatocellular carcinoma. Four are currently alive (1 lung, 1 colon, the prostate, and the cervical cancer sufferer) including the patient with SCC in the lung who underwent lobectomy. In all others the tumor metastatized swiftly, leading to death.

Skin malignancies (SCC, basal cell carcinoma [BCC], and keratoacanthomas) are extremely common posttransplant and should be biopsied and treated early. Cyclosporine probably increases the risk of skin malignancies further. Frequent dermatological review is required for those with multiple solar keratotic lesions. High UV protection sunscreen (Factor 15) is recommended to limit the contribution of UV irradiation.

Preexistent Malignancies

Since the use of cyclosporine at Stanford, seven patients with a history of prior malignancy have undergone transplantation. These included 4 with treated lymphoma (2 Hogdkins, 1 non-Hodgkin, and 1 Burkitts lymphoma—disease-free intervals were 10, 12, 9, and 6 years respectively), 1 with retinoblastoma (2-year disease-free interval), and 1 with acute lymphoblastic leukemia (10-year disease-free). All patients were transplanted for adriamycin cardiotoxicity, and in none of these cases has tumor recurred posttransplant. The seventh patient was a man who had undergone hemicolectomy for bowel carcinoma 2 years prior to heart transplantation for ischemic cardiomyopathy, but tumor recurred early posttransplant and caused death.

Chronic Renal Failure

Renal impairment posttransplant is common with cyclosporine based immunosuppression and is due, in the main, to dose and time-related nephrotoxicity secondary to cyclosporine. In some patients, prerenal azotemia pretransplant does not reverse fully with the establishment of a normal cardiac output and this contributes to renal failure posttransplant. Mean serum creatinine at 1 year in recent patient cohorts is around 1.6 mg/dL and generally increases slowly with time.

Etiology

The mechanism of cyclosporine nephrotoxicity remains unclear but appears to occur in three general forms:

1. Transient Acute Renal Failure—This is most common in the first weeks of therapy with cyclosporine or immediately following initiation of therapy. It is usually brief and at least partially reversible after the dosage of cyclosporine is reduced. The mechanism may include increased renal vascular resistance with increased sympathetic nervous activity, efferent glomerular arteriolar vasoconstriction and activation of the renin-angiotensin system.
2. Protracted Renal Failure—Renal failure may become protracted beyond 1 week. Histologic changes include increased numbers of mitochondria in the proximal convoluted tubule, vacuolization of the tubular lining cells, and a mild arteriolopathy with marked interstitial fibrosis.
3. Chronic Nephropathy—Virtually all patients on cyclosporine have some degree of chronic renal impairment, usually in the vicinity of 50% reduction in glomerular filtration rate and renal plasma flow, mild proteinuria, and evidence of tubular dysfunction on testing. The chronic renal impairment associated with cyclosporine is generally progressive. Histologic changes consist of tubular atrophy and interstitial fibrosis, focal segmental glomerular sclerosis, and focal arteriolar hyalinosis.

Results

At Stanford to date, five cyclosporine treated patients have required long-term dialysis for progressive renal impairment. Four of these subsequently underwent successful renal transplantation.

Prophylaxis

Minimization of renal failure involves avoidance of diuretic and other nephrotoxic therapy posttransplant. All usual nephrotoxic drugs are considerably more detrimental when used in combination with cyclosporine. Careful monitoring must be employed when using agents that interfere with the metabolism of cyclosporine and lead to elevated serum and tissue levels (see Chapter 6). Deterioration of renal function in this setting is often not reversible.

Hypertension

Etiology

The occurrence of systemic hypertension has been the rule rather than the exception since the introduction of cyclosporine. It is uncertain whether the hypertension contributes to chronic renal impairment or whether the renal impairment contributes to hypertension (or both). Plasma volume is expanded by around 15% and there is some evidence for poor adaptation of the renin-angiotensin system to this fluid retention. Elevated circulating catecholamine levels and treatment with corticosteroids may also play a role.

Incidence

By 12 months posttransplant, more than 80% of cardiac transplant recipients of all ages require antihypertensive therapy. The incidence of hypertension does not fall significantly even when steroids can be discontinued.

Management

Hypertension following cardiac transplantation may be extremely resistant to treatment, often requiring polypharmacy to achieve the target blood pressure of <140/90. Malignant levels (e.g., of 170/110) are not uncommon. Systemic hypertension may cause headaches and flushing and occasionally in the early postoperative period, may cause seizures (particularly in children). The usual signs such as retinal vascular changes and proteinuria (>1 gm/day) are rarely present. Home monitoring of blood pressure by the patient or family is desirable to maintain satisfactory control.

Side effects of anti-hypertensive treatment are the same as seen in other patients. Particularly common complaints are listed below under the specific agent.

Nifedipine: Useful in the postoperative setting sublingually for rapid reduction of blood pressure. Chronic administration is often associated with peripheral edema and flushing due to marked vasodilation in the presence of an already expanded plasma volume.

Verapamil: Not often utilized, limited experience with this agent to date.

Diltiazem: Not particularly effective in this population. During a trial of diltiazem for prophylaxis of CAD, there has been no reduction in the antihypertensive requirements of those randomized to diltiazem. Diltiazem reduces the metabolism of cyclosporine such that the dose of cyclosporine can be halved within the first week of commencing diltiazem, a change leading to substantial cost reduction.

Beta-Blockers: Commonly used. Metoprolol and atenolol are effective. Usual side effects are not uncommon. These agents should not be used in those with impaired systolic function (e.g., left ventricular ejection fraction <40%) as they can precipitate cardiac failure.

Hydralazine: A useful agent, well tolerated, and inexpensive. Maximal doses should not exceed 50 mg tid because of concern about development of a lupus-like syndrome at doses above 150 mg/day.

Prazosin: An effective agent but often not tolerated in doses above 3 mg tid because of postural hypotension.

Clonidine: Useful and well tolerated. Transdermal patches provide long-term, smooth blood pressure control.

ACE Inhibitors: Well tolerated in maximal doses (enalapril 15 mg bid, captopril 50 mg tid), effective agents. These drugs may rarely potentiate cyclosporine nephrotoxicity.

Diuretics: Not for use in this population group because of enhancement of the nephrotoxic effects of cyclosporine. In the main, the only patients who require diuretics on a regular basis are those with systolic dysfunction where these agents are needed for control of heart failure. Avoid where possible.

Summary: First line agents:
1. Hydralazine
2. Captopril/Enalapril
3. Prazosin
4. Beta-Blockers
5. Clonidine.

A combination of these is often required, working up to maximal doses of each before introducing the next agent.

Hyperlipidemia

Prevalence

Elevation of both cholesterol and triglycerides is highly prevalent following cardiac transplantation. Hypercholesterolemia is related to use of cyclosporine (ill defined mechanism) and prednisone and correlates with weight gain posttransplant. Of those with prior ischemic heart disease, 50% demonstrate hypercholesterolemia and 10% have hypertriglyceridemia at 12-months posttransplant. Of those with underlying idiopathic dilated cardiomyopathy, 33% display hypercholesterolemia at 12 months and 8% have elevated triglyceride levels. Elevation in total cholesterol consists of 15% mean increase in LDL, 56% increase in HDL, with VLDL 28% below normal. Hyperlipidemia does not usually require treatment before 3-months posttransplant.

Implications

There is some evidence that elevated cholesterol may contribute to more rapid development of graft atherosclerosis. Elevations of cholesterol and triglycerides are associated with the development of proximal and mid-vessel discrete coronary artery stenoses and elevated LDL cholesterol and triglycerides with concentric distal disease. It is recommended that lipid elevations be treated in the expectation that the rate of peripheral vascular disease, and possibly TxCAD may be reduced long-term.

Treatment

Diet: Cholesterol restricted diet (<35% of energy from fat, cholesterol <300 mg/day). Achieve and maintain ideal body weight for height.

Probucol: Well tolerated; few side effects. No noted interference with cyclosporine. Agent of first choice.

Cholestyramine: May reduce the absorption of cyclosporine. Monitoring of cyclosporine levels required if this agent is used. Average 11% fall in serum cholesterol.

Clofibrate: Concern because of increased cardiovascular risk profile in general population studies. Rarely used.

Nicotinic Acid: Effective. Often poorly tolerated in therapeutic doses (flushing, abdominal cramps).

Gemfibrozil: Moderately effective, reasonably tolerated.

HMG CoA Reductase Inhibitors: High risk of rhabdomyolysis and resultant renal failure when used in normal doses in combination with cyclosporine. Mevolinin may be used in low doses without this complication but close monitoring of creatinine, CPK, and cyclosporine should be performed for the duration of therapy.

Results

Overall Survival

Overall actuarial survival rates with the current triple drug immunosuppressive protocol using cyclosporine, azathioprine, and prednisone at Stanford are 82% at 1 year, 61% at 5 years, and 41% at 10 years after transplantation (Figure 2). These survival rates represent substantial improvement over the results achieved before the clinical availability of cyclosporine (approximately 20 percentage points at each time interval). Figure 2 also illustrates the dismal prognosis of patients officially selected for transplantation at Stanford, but who died before a suitable donor became available. Such patients do not, of course, provide a formally adequate "control" group, but their very limited survival serves to illustrate the severity of cardiac disease present in patients selected for transplantation in our program.

In a recent analysis of the Stanford cardiac transplantation experience (496 patients) in the cyclosporine era, overall operative mortality (defined as death in the hospital posttransplant, even beyond 30 days) was 7.9% ± 1.3% (70% confidence intervals). The major causes of early death were infection (49%), pulmonary hypertension (15%), nonspecific graft failure (10%), and rejection (8%). Multivariate logistic regression analysis revealed that peroperative higher pulmonary vascular resistance and female gender were the only independent predictors of early death. Although pediatric age was a univariate predictor of early death (operative mortality

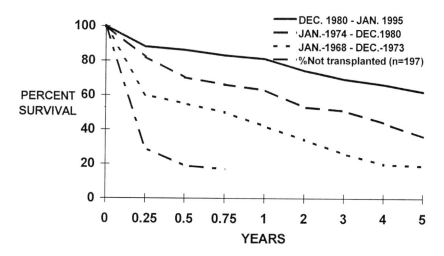

Figure 2. Actuarial survival according to period of transplantation. Dec 1980–Jan 1995—Cyclosporine based immunosuppression. Jan 1974–Dec 1980—Azathioprine, prednisone, and rabbit antithymocyte globulin (RATG), plus transvenous endomyocardial biopsy. Jan 1968–Dec 1973—Azathioprine, prednisone, and various crude antilymphocyte serum preparations.

15% ± 5% for patients under 18 years of age compared with 7% ± 1.3% for those over age 18), this factor dropped out of the multivariate equation when pulmonary vascular resistance was considered.

Although most deaths occur early (within the first few months post-transplant), there is continuing attrition (approximately 5% per year), attributable largely to late infection (34%), transplant coronary disease (18%), and late acute cellular rejection (14%). Cox model multivariate analysis of the Stanford cyclosporine experience revealed that older recipient age was the most important independent risk factor for late death, but transplant year and particular immunosuppressive protocol (e.g., OKT3) did not independently affect survival. Pediatric patients have higher early mortality, as noted above, but improved long-term survival. Actuarial analysis also showed a trend of reduced survival for patients in their sixth decade of life, but this did not achieve statistical significance. The development of CMV infection has been shown to limit long-term survival (Figure 3A) and to be associated with higher rates of death from TxCAD (Figure 3B).

Rehabilitation

The goal of cardiac transplantation is not only to prolong life, but also to rehabilitate patients to an active lifestyle with good quality of life.

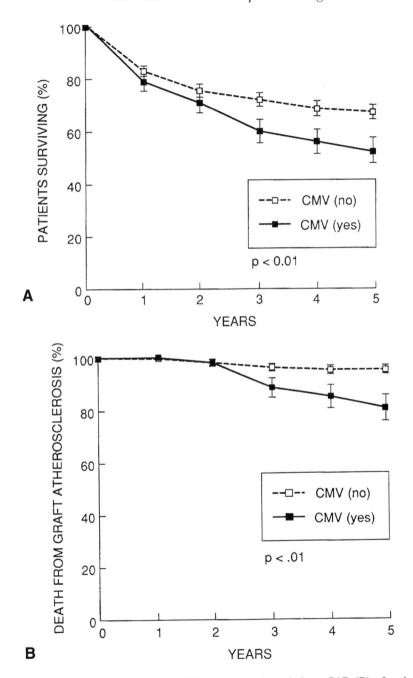

Figure 3A and 3B. Actuarial survival (A) and rates of death from CAD (B) of recipients with and without postoperative CMV infection. (Reproduced with permission from Grattan, et al).

Numerous studies indicate that the latter is usually achievable. Whether patients return to work or not relates to several factors—stability and duration of prior employment, and whether a position has been held open. A common reason given for persisting unemployment is unwillingness on the part of potential employers to hire cardiac transplant recipients.

Only under exceptional circumstances, involving high risk occupations, must consideration be given to a change in the nature of employment (e.g., microbiology technicians, abattoir workers, professional contact sport players). Unless there are ongoing complications, recipients may return to work as early as 3-months posttransplant.

Of 385 1-year survivors recently analyzed at Stanford, 59% had returned to work, full-time study, or child care, 17% were voluntarily retired, 15% were unemployed for a variety of reasons (unable to find work, voluntary unemployment, disability insurance), and only 9% were medically disabled.

Compliance

A minority of patients (most commonly adolescents), demonstrate poor compliance with immunosuppressive therapy. Cessation of immunosuppression predictably results in graft and patient loss within days to weeks. Psychological counseling, especially of adolescent patients, may therefore be extremely important.

Cigarette smoking and illicit drugs are clearly contraindicated posttransplant.

Alcohol may be taken in moderation (20 gm ethanol/day—i.e., 2 beverages/day) but higher intake may potentially lead to hepatic abnormalities with fluctuation in cyclosporine metabolism. Under dire circumstances, cyclosporine may be mixed and taken with alcohol, although adherence to one vehicle (either milk or orange juice) is more prudent.

Selected References

1. Alonso P, Starek P, Minich R. Studies on the pathogenesis of atheroarteriosclerosis induced in rabbit cardiac allografts by the synergy of graft rejection and hypercholesterolemia. Am J Pathol 1977;87:415–435.
2. Anderson J, Schroeder J. Effects of probucol on hyperlipidemic patients with cardiac allografts. J Cardiovasc Pharmacol 1979;1:3:353–365.
3. Ballantyne CM, Jones PH, Payton-Ross C, et al. Hyperlipidemia following heart transplantation: Natural history and intervention with mevinolin (lovastatin). Transplant Proc 1987;19:(Suppl):60–62.

4. Beiber C, Hunt S, Schwinn A. Complications in long-term survivors of cardiac transplantation. Transpl Proc 1981;13:207–211.

5. Bellett M, Cabrol C, Sassano P, et al. Systemic hypertension after cardiac transplantation: Effect of cyclosporine on the renin-angiotensin system. Am J Cardiol 1985;56:927–931.

6. East C, Alivizatos P, Grundy S, et al. Rhabdomyolysis in patients receiving lovastatin after cardiac transplantation. N Engl J Med 1988;318:1:47–48.

7. Frazier O, Macris M, Lammermeier D, et al. Heart transplantation in 234 patients: Review of the Texas Heart Institute six year experience. Transplant Proc 1989;21:1:2489.

8. Gao S, Hunt SA, Schroder JS. Accelerated transplant coronary artery disease. Semin Thorac Cardiovasc Surg 1990;2:241–249.

9. Gao S, Schroeder J, Alderman E, et al. Clinical and laboratory correlates of accelerated coronary artery disease in the cardiac transplant patient. Circulation 1987;76:5:V56-V61.

10. Gao S, Schroeder J, Hunt S, et al. Retransplantation for severe accelerated coronary artery disease in heart transplant recipients. Am J Cardiol 1988;62:876–881.

11. Grattan MT, Moreno-Cabral CE, Starnes VA, et al. Cytomegalovirus infection is associated with cardiac allograft rejection and atherosclerosis. JAMA 1989;261: 24:3561–3566.

12. Hess M, Hastillo A, Mohanakumar T, et al. Accelerated atherosclerosis in cardiac transplantation: Role of cytotoxic B-cell antibodies and hyperlipidemia. Circulation 1983;68(Suppl 2):II94–101.

13. Keogh A, Simons L, Spratt P, et al. Hyperlipidemia following cardiac transplantation. J Heart Transplant 1988;7:171–175.

14. Kriett JM, Kaye MP. The registry of the international society for heart transplantation: Seventh official report—1990. J Heart Transplant 1990;9:323–330.

15. Lurie K, Billingham M, Jamieson S, et al. Pathogenesis and prevention of graft arteriosclerosis in an experimental heart transplant model. Transplantation 1981;31:41–47.

16. McDonald K, Rector T, Braunlin E, et al. Association of coronary artery disease in cardiac transplant recipients with CMV infection. Am J Cardiol 1989;64: 359–362.

17. Myers BD, Ross J, Newton L, et al. Cyclosporine associated chronic nephropathy. N Engl J Med 1984;311:699–705.

18. Neild GH. Cyclosporin nephrotoxicity. Semin Thorac Cardiovasc Surg 1990;2: 198–203.

19. Norman D, Illingworth D, Munson J, et al. Myolysis and acute renal failure in a heart transplant recipient receiving lovostatin. N Engl J Med 1988;318:1:46–48.

20. Penn I. Cancers following cyclosporine therapy. Transplant Proc 1987;19:1: 2211–2213.

21. Penn I. Problems of cancer in organ transplantation. J Heart Transplant 1982;2:1:71–77.

22. Samuelson RG, Hunt SA, Schroeder JS. Functional and social rehabilitation of heart transplant recipients under age thirty. Scand J Thorac Cardiovasc Surg 1984;18:97–103.

23. Sarris GE, Moore KA, Schroeder JS, et al. Cardiac transplantation: The Stanford experience in the cyclosporine era. J Thorac Cardiovasc Surg 1994;108:240–252.

24. Sarris GE, Smith JA, Bernstein D, et al. Pediatric cardiac transplantation. The Stanford experience. Circulation 1994;90:II-51–II-55.
25. Schroeder JS, Gao SZ, Alderman EL, et al. A preliminary study of diltiazem in the prevention of coronary artery disease in heart-transplant recipients. N Engl J Med 1993;328:164–170.
26. Smith JA, Ribakove GH, Hunt SA, et al. Cardiac retransplantation: The 25 year experience at a single institution. J Heart Lung Transplant 1995;14:832–839.
27. Starzl TE, Nalesnik MA, Porter K, et al. Reversibility of lymphomas and lymphoproliferative lesions developing under cyclosporin-steroid therapy. Lancet 1984;17:583–587.
28. Taylor D, Thompson J, Hastillo A, et al. Hyperlipidemia after heart transplantation. J Heart Transplant 1989;8:209–213.
29. Thompson J, Eich P, Ko D, et al. Hypercholesterolemia as a marker of early coronary artery disease post cardiac transplantation. J Heart Transplant 1987;4:167.
30. Valantine H, Pinto FJ, St. Goar FG, et al. Intracoronary ultrasound imaging in heart transplant recipients: The Stanford experience. J Heart Lung Transplant 1992;11:S60–S64.
31. Wilkinson A, Smith J, Hunsicker L. Increased frequency of posttransplant lymphomas in patients treated with cyclosporine, azathioprine and prednisone. Transplantation 1989;47:293–296.

Chapter 9

Evaluation and Selection of Recipients and Donors for Heart-Lung and Lung Transplantation

Sara E. Marshall, M.B., B.S., Ph.D., MRCP,
Patrick M. McCarthy, M.D., Mordechai R. Kramer, M.D.,
Norman J. Lewiston, M.D., Vaughn A. Starnes, M.D.,
Edward B. Stinson, M.D., James Theodore, M.D.

The success of heart-lung and lung transplantation depends in large part upon the selection of appropriate candidates. In our experience patients who are most likely to benefit are those who, while terminally ill, continue to have the strength and stamina to maintain a relatively active lifestyle. Only in exceptional cases will hospitalized, critically ill patients be considered for transplant candidacy, and when selecting patients for these procedures it is important to be continually reminded that desperate clinical situations are not, in themselves, indications for transplantation. To help in patient evaluation, we have drawn up a list of criteria and contraindications for patient selection based on the Stanford experience. As our experience increases, these criteria may vary.

Indications for Heart-Lung and Lung Transplantation

Indications and Requirements for Transplantation

End-stage Pulmonary or Cardiopulmonary Disease

Any patient with end-stage cardiopulmonary or pulmonary disease (Table 1) with the capacity for full rehabilitation can be considered for

From: Smith JA, McCarthy PM, Sarris GE, Stinson EB, Reitz BA (eds.): The Stanford Manual of Cardiopulmonary Transplantation. Futura Publishing Co., Inc., Armonk, NY, 1996.

Table 1

Diseases for Which Cardiopulmonary Transplantation has Been Performed

Heart-Lung Transplantation
  Primary pulmonary hypertension
  Pulmonary hypertension secondary to thromboembolic disease
  Eisenmenger's syndrome (ASD, VSD, PDA, Truncus, other complex anomalies)
  Cardiomyopathy with pulmonary hypertension
  Emphysema
  Cystic fibrosis
  Bronchiectasis
  Histiocytosis X
  Asbestosis
  Bronchiolitis obliterans organizing pneumonia (BOOP)
  Posttransplant obliterative bronchiolitis
  Sarcoidosis
  Desquamative interstitial pneumonitis
  Lymphangioleiomyomatosis

Single-Lung Transplant
  Idiopathic pulmonary fibrosis
  Sarcoidosis
  Primary pulmonary hypertension
  Eisenmenger's syndrome (ASD, PDA, small VSD)
  Emphysema
  Posttransplant obliterative bronchiolitis
  Asbestosis
  Bronchopulmonary dysplasia

Double-Lung Transplant (Bilateral Sequential)
  Cystic fibrosis
  Bronchioectasis
  Emphysema
  Primary pulmonary hypertension
  Pulmonary hypertension with ventricular septal defect

transplantation, although obviously not all will be suitable. All patients should have a life expectancy of <2 years, and should be New York Heart Association (NYHA) Class III or IV.

Otherwise Vigorous and Free of Systemic Disease

It is of the utmost importance that candidates should be in otherwise good health and be without other serious medical illness.

Emotionally Stable with Firm Commitment
to the Idea of Transplantation

Transplantation demands that candidates must have the emotional stability to confront their own mortality, and the strength to withstand the uncertainty of the waiting period. They must have a commitment to the idea of transplantation and a willingness to be completely compliant with rigorous and intrusive medical regimens. Patients with a history of psychiatric disturbance tend to cope poorly with the demands of both the waiting period and the early posttransplant period.

Contraindications to Heart-Lung and Lung Transplantation (Table 2)

Absolute Contraindications

Significant Systemic or Multisystem Disease. At this time transplantation cannot be offered to patients with significant systemic disease. The presence of multi-organ involvement limits the possibility of full recovery and furthermore may compromise the function of the newly transplanted organ(s).

Active Infection. In view of the need to heavily immunosuppress patients after cardiopulmonary or pulmonary transplantation, patients with active extrapulmonary sites of infection are not considered candidates for trans-

---

Table 2
Contraindications to Heart-Lung and Lung Transplantation

Significant systemic or multisystem disease
Active or systemic infection
Significant hepatic disease
Significant renal disease
Cachexia or obesity
Corticosteroid therapy
Current cigarette smoking
Psychiatric illness
History of drug abuse
Previous cardiac or thoracic surgery (may be considered on a case-by-case basis)
Age >45 years (heart-lung transplant), or >55 years (lung transplant)

plantation. Successful heart-lung and bilateral sequential lung transplantation can be offered to those with chronic infection confined to the respiratory tract (i.e., chronic bronchiectasis and cystic fibrosis [CF]). Single-lung transplantation should not, however ever be performed in such patients as infection may "spill" from the remaining native lung into the transplanted lung.

Significant Hepatic Disease.   In view of the hepatotoxicity of many of the posttransplant medications, normal hepatic function is required in all transplant candidates. The only exception to this occurs in those patients who have abnormal liver function consequent to right ventricular failure. Even in this group (usually patients with pulmonary hypertension), those who have a total bilirubin of >2.1 mg% despite maximal diuresis tend to be at high risk of perioperative complications. These include coagulopathies, hepatic encephalopathy, infection, and poor wound healing. Furthermore, impaired hepatic function may impair clearance of cyclosporine with consequent cyclosporine nephrotoxicity.

Significant Renal Disease.   Adequate renal reserve must be present at the time of operation to avoid possible renal failure as a consequence of cyclosporine nephrotoxicity. All patients should have a preoperative serum creatinine of <1.5 mg/dL and a 24-hour creatinine clearance >50 mL/min. Occasional exceptions to this rule consist of patients with severe pulmonary hypertension and subsequent poor renal perfusion in whom creatinine clearances of >35 mL/min may be acceptable once intrinsic renal disease has been excluded. Improvement in cardiac output postoperatively may result in dramatic improvement in renal function in this group of patients.

Current Cigarette Smoking.   Patients who continue to smoke cigarettes despite terminal lung disease cannot be considered for transplantation because of the assumed detrimental effects of smoking on the transplanted heart and lung. We insist that all patients abstain from cigarette smoking for at least 2 years prior to consideration for transplantation.

History of Illicit Drug Use.   Patients with a history of drug abuse should not be considered for transplantation. In rare circumstances, if a psychological evaluation indicates emotional stability and if abstention from illicit drug use for 2 years can be conclusively demonstrated (e.g., by repeated urine tests), such patients may be evaluated.

Relative Contraindications

Previous Cardiac or Thoracic Surgery.   In the early years of heart-lung transplantation many of the early postoperative deaths were attributed to bleeding problems caused by chest wall adhesions. Previous cardiothoracic surgery, therefore, became an absolute contraindication to transplantation. In the past, chest tube insertion or open lung biopsy were also contraindications to transplantation. With greater experience and improved surgical techniques, patients with either previous thoracotomies or median sternotomies can now be considered on a case by case basis. A greater range of procedures are now available (such as single-lung transplant, single-lung transplant with cardiac repair, bilateral sequential lung transplant, and single lung and heart transplant as well as the more conventional heart-lung transplant), and patients are evaluated individually for the most suitable operation.

While adhesions and postoperative bleeding remain a significant risk, patients with previous procedures may now be considered for transplantation. Chemical or surgical pleurodesis remain absolute contraindications to heart-lung transplant.

Age.   The current upper age limit for heart-lung transplantation at Stanford is 45 with one exception: patients with emphysema are considered eligible up to age 50. The upper limit for single and bilateral sequential lung transplantation is 55. However, these are guidelines only and absolute limits may be waived in certain cases, with great emphasis being placed on the physiologic condition of the patient. There is no lower age limit for transplantation.

Peptic Ulcer Disease.   Gastrointestinal problems are very common postoperatively and a history of peptic ulcer disease is a relative contraindication to transplantation. However, if this is the only contraindication to surgery, candidacy may in some cases be considered if active ulcer disease can be excluded.

Corticosteroids.   Corticosteroids have been implicated as a contributory cause of tracheal and bronchial dehiscence in the early postoperative period. For this reason, patients should be tapered off all corticosteroids prior to transplant candidacy. Some patients may have to be intermittently withdrawn from the active list during exacerbations of their disease if steroid therapy is instituted, and reinstated once their steroids have been tapered. Steroid withdrawal requires careful tapering of steroid dose, with or without the introduction of alternative therapy (usually cyclophosphamide for pulmonary fibrosis patients).

Nutritional Status.   Despite the presence of severe underlying cardiopulmonary or pulmonary disease, the overall physical condition of prospective transplant candidates should be relatively good, with preservation of muscle mass, good muscle tone, and sound nutrition. Activity is encouraged and preoperative physical therapy may be required (in some cases).

Patients showing signs of cachexia represent poor operative candidates although they may respond to measures such as gastrostomy feeding. Marked obesity is also a relative contraindication as poor postoperative mobilization and impaired diaphragmatic function may complicate recovery, and weight control is particularly difficult once steroid immunosuppression is instituted. Therefore, we prefer candidates to be within 25% of their ideal weight for height, sex, and race.

Anticipating the "Transplant Window"

Anticipating the most appropriate time for transplantation is extremely difficult. With an average wait of 12 months for our heart-lung waiting list we try to select recipients who have a life expectancy of no more than 2 years. We term the period of time during which a patient is sick enough to require transplantation and well enough for it to be performed with a high probability of success the "transplant window" (Figure 1). Obviously, identifying this period is an inaccurate art, but certain pointers have been defined that may be helpful.

Natural History of the Disease and Previous Course

Knowledge of the natural history of a particular disease can help in anticipating its future course. Of even greater importance is the progression of disease in individual patients. Many patients can identify a turning point in their disease, often a significant event such as a syncopal episode, infection, or episode of hemoptysis, which is followed by an accelerated course. Identification of such turning points can help in choosing the appropriate time for placing a patient on the active waiting list.

"TRANSPLANT WINDOW"

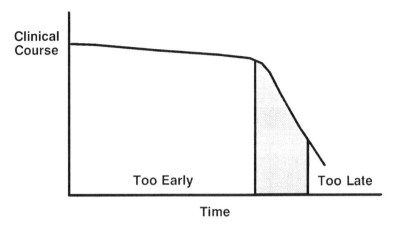

Figure 1. The transplant window: when is the right time for transplantation?

Functional Status

Exercise Tolerance

The functional status of a patient is of particular importance in patient assessment. Criteria such as the ability to climb one flight of stairs or walk one city block are given great credence. Rate of change in exercise tolerance is especially important as it is a useful predictor for future decline. We do not usually formally exercise patients, relying more on personal and collateral history in our assessment of exercise capability.

Pulmonary Function

Sequential pulmonary function studies may be useful in monitoring the course of patients with obstructive lung disease. Increasing supplemental oxygen requirements may also be a clue indicating declining status in patients with primary parenchymal disease such as pulmonary fibrosis.

Deteriorating Cardiac or Hepatic Function

Increasing right ventricular dysfunction, usually manifest by increased requirement for diuretics or a rising serum bilirubin, is of particular importance in patients with pulmonary hypertension. In this group of patients, these findings often herald rapid deterioration, even though it may be asymptomatic at first. Hepatic function is therefore monitored every 2–3 months in patients in whom transplantation is being considered but not actively pursued.

Life-Threatening Arrhythmias and Hemoptysis

A history of life-threatening arrhythmias, or syncope, would merit consideration for early candidacy, as would the onset of hemoptysis.

Patient Evaluation

Referral

Only approximately 10% of those about whom we receive inquiries are considered suitable for interview, and in general only 50% of these are accepted onto the active transplant list. Thus patient selection is a process of exclusion, and only a very small minority of those referred will ever get transplanted.

The referral process usually begins with a letter of inquiry from the patient's physician to the transplant team. It is expeditious to include in this letter enough clinical information for the reviewer to determine whether there are any absolute contraindications to the surgery. If there are not and the patient appears to be a suitable candidate, the referring physician is sent an application packet requesting additional medical and psychosocial information. Once this material is received it is again reviewed and, if appropriate, the candidate is invited to come to Stanford for an evaluation, which usually takes about 3 days.

Interview

This interview includes a full history and physical examination, a discussion about transplantation in general during which potential risks and benefits are outlined as objectively as possible, and a dialogue about the details of transplantation in a patient's specific situation. A candidate is usually seen by two or more members of the evaluating team to try to maximize objective assessment.

Patients are requested to have routine investigations performed on the day prior to interview (Table 3). These are therefore available at the interview and help identify potential problems. Patients are actively encouraged to bring family members with them for the assessment.

If a candidate appears to be suitable and is interested in continuing to pursue the transplant option, more blood is drawn for tissue typing, viral serologies, and other relevant studies (Table 3). Depending on the anticipated procedure, other investigations are scheduled as appropriate (see below). Candidates also meet with the medical social worker to obtain a pager and to help organize air transport if appropriate, as patients must guarantee that they can be at Stanford within 2–1/2 hours of receiving notice of a donor organ.

In some patients, problems will be identified that, while currently ex-

---

Table 3
Pretransplant Investigations

Initial Screening Studies
   Chest film: PA and lateral
   ECG
   CBC with differential, platelet count and reticulocyte count
   Blood type and Rh antibody screen
   Coagulation screen with bleeding time
   Serum electrolytes, renal panel and hepatic panel
   Serum protein electrophoresis
   Rheumatoid factor and FANA
   Full urinalysis
   Sputum culture and sensitivity (include fungal and TB cultures)

Post Acceptance Studies
   Viral screen including HIV, Hepatitis B, Hepatitis C, HSV, VZ, EBV, Adenovirus
     and CMV
   Complement fixation for coccidioidomycosis and histoplasmosis
   Toxoplasma titer
   HLA typing, HLA-DR typing, transplant antibody screen
   T lymphocyte subsets for transplant monitoring
   Quantitative immunoglobulins
   Indirect plasma lipoprotein fractionation
   Full pulmonary function testing
   24-hour creatinine clearance

(Echocardiography, Holter monitoring, MUGA scan or MRI, cardiac catheterization, etc., as appropriate)

cluding a patient from transplantation, do not appear insurmountable. Such problems include obesity or low weight, and reversible liver or renal dysfunction. Recommendations will be made to the referring physician and patients reassessed once these problems have been addressed.

Others may be placed "on hold" for review at a later date if it is felt that they are potential candidates but have not yet entered their "transplant window".

Once Listed for "Active Status"

During the waiting period we encourage patients to continue regular contact with their primary care physicians and to notify the transplant team of any hospitalizations or changes in medication. We review patients every 3–6 months in the evaluation clinic and maintain frequent contact with their physicians. Unfortunately at present 20% of patients on the waiting list die before a suitable donor can be found.

Choosing the Most Appropriate Procedure

The Choices

There are two broad groups of transplant options: the single-lung procedures and the heart-lung/bilateral sequential lung procedures.

Single-lung transplantation was initially only offered to patients with fibrotic lung disease, but has since been adapted for patients with chronic obstructive pulmonary disease (COPD) and those with pulmonary hypertension, both idiopathic and secondary to congenital heart disease. There are significant advantages to the single-lung transplant procedures in appropriate candidates. Most importantly, donor availability is greater and waiting times are therefore shorter than for heart-lung transplants. There are three main reasons for this. Some donors will have sustained damage to one lung and will therefore be unsuitable for heart-lung transplantation but the nondamaged lung can be used for single-lung transplantation. Second, Status I heart transplant recipients have priority over heart-lung transplant recipients and "compete" for the scarce donor hearts. Finally, one heart-lung donor can provide separate grafts for three transplants—a heart, right lung, and left lung. Other advantages of single-lung transplantation include shorter postoperative recovery time and in-hospital stay. The absence of cardiac replacement also means that those problems specific to the heart, such as heart rejection, graft coronary artery disease, and cardiac denervation do not arise.

The heart-lung and "domino" operation is an option in patients requiring bilateral lung replacement (e.g., patients with CF and bronchiectasis) with essentially normal cardiac function. In this procedure, the explanted heart of a heart-lung recipient is transplanted into a patient waiting for a cardiac transplant.

Double-lung transplantation has also been used in the treatment of patients with bilateral pulmonary sepsis (CF and bronchiectasis) or COPD with essentially normal hearts. While double-lung transplantation has the advantage of retaining the native heart, the "classic" en-block double-lung transplant operation is associated with significant airway problems and has been abandoned by most centers in favor of the bilateral sequential lung transplant procedure, which has not been plagued by bronchial healing complications. The choice between heart-lung "domino" transplantation and bilateral sequential lung transplantation currently remains a question of center preference and a focus of further clinical investigation, although the current United Network for Organ Sharing criteria have further limited the number of heart-lung grafts becoming available (donors are not offered for heart-lung recipients unless there is no Status I heart recipient).

Transplantation of the heart and one lung has been performed in several patients in Paris. It has been suggested that it is a suitable operation for those in whom unilateral extensive pleural adhesions contraindicate cardiopulmonary replacement. Although there is no experience with this procedure at Stanford, our group would consider it in carefully selected patients.

How to Choose?

In Table 4 the most suitable procedures for different diseases are outlined. In general, it should be remembered that infective pulmonary disease requires transplantation of both lungs because of the risk of cross infection; and, severe concurrent cardiac disease, whether primary, secondary, or unrelated to pulmonary disease, requires cardiac replacement. Preferences of individual surgical teams will also determine the range of options available.

Table 4
Options for Transplantation

A. Heart-Lung Transplantation
   Eisenmenger's syndrome with "uncorrectable" congenital heart disease (e.g., truncus arteriosus, AV canal, TGA)
   Other types of Eisenmenger's syndrome with severe right ventricular decompensation
   Primary pulmonary hypertension with severe right ventricular decompensation and/or cardiomyopathy
   Concurrent cardiac and pulmonary disease (e.g., coronary artery disease, malignant arrhythmias)
B. Heart-Lung and Domino Transplant
   Cystic fibrosis/bronchiectasis (in the absence of cardiac decompensation)
   Emphysema/COPD
C. Double-Lung Transplant (Bilateral sequential lung transplant)
   (En-block double-lung transplant not used at Stanford)
   Cystic fibrosis/bronchiectasis
   Emphysema/COPD
   Primary pulmonary hypertension without severe right ventricular decompensation
D. Single-Lung Transplant
   Pulmonary fibrosis
   Emphysema
   Pulmonary hypertension without significant right heart dysfunction
   Posttransplant obliterative bronchiolitis
   Bronchopulmonary dysplasia
E. Single-Lung Transplant with Cardiac Repair
   Eisenmenger's syndrome with correctable congenital heart disease
      Right lung transplant: ASD, small VSD
      Left lung transplant: PDA
F. Single-Lung and Heart Transplant
   Disease requiring both cardiac and pulmonary replacement in patients with previous thoracotomy and extensive pleural adhesions

Evaluating Candidates for Single-Lung Transplantation

Single-lung transplantation was pioneered as a treatment for fibrotic lung disease, but has since been adapted for a variety of other conditions. The evaluation of patients for single-lung transplantation is essentially the same as for heart-lung transplantation. Exceptions are that a history of previous cardiothoracic operation is not a contraindication to single-lung transplantation; and, as the surgery itself is usually less onerous, an older group of patients can be considered for this procedure (up to age 55).

Table 5
Preoperative Evaluation of Patients with Pulmonary Hypertension Assessing Suitability for Single-Lung Transplantation

Investigation	Indication	Criteria for Single-Lung Transplantation
Echo Doppler	All candidates	Good left ventricular function contractility, moderate or less right ventricular dysfunction, no more than mild to moderate mitral regurgitation
Saline contrast (Bubble) study	Patients with PPH: To exclude any previously undiagnosed intracardiac shunting	A positive bubble study should be followed by cardiac catheterization in patients with previously unsuspected intracardiac shunt
Radionucleotide scan (MUGA)	All candidates	RVEF >20% LVEF >40% These values may be inaccurate in patients with intracardiac defects should be corroborated with cardiac catheterization
Holter monitor	Patients with a history of palpitations or arrhythmias	Absent or minimal ventricular arrhythmias
Cardiac catheterization	Patients with Eisenmenger's syndrome to define the exact nature of the cardiac defect; in patients at high risk for coronary artery disease, (age >50, history of cigarette smoking, strong family history, hypertension, hyperlipidemia)	Good right and left ventricular function dysfunction; no coronary disease.

Pulmonary Hypertension

In our early experience, patients with both primary and secondary pulmonary hypertension have tolerated single-lung transplant well, and in some patients with Eisenmenger's physiology transplantation can be combined with repair of the cardiac defect. Adequacy of cardiac function is the most important factor in determining whether a patient will tolerate this procedure. Some patients whom we currently think require cardiac replacement include: those with significant cardiomegaly on clinical examination or chest film; those with hepatomegaly, rising serum bilirubin, or increasing diuretic requirement; and those with a history of myocardial infarction or malignant arrhythmias. In patients in whom the situation is less clear cut, preoperative evaluation includes an echo-Doppler and MUGA scan and when indicated 24-hour Holter monitoring, bubble study, or cardiac catheterization (Table 5). The extent of cardiac dysfunction that will be reversible following single-lung transplant is an active area of research. The criteria in the table are conservative and most likely will be modified as experience increases (see Chapter 12, Future Directions).

COPD/Emphysema

Although both single and bilateral sequential lung transplants have been performed on patients with severe emphysema/COPD, the optimal procedure has not been determined. Although pulmonary function tests are better after bilateral transplantation, there is no clear advantage in terms of exercise capacity. Although single lung transplantation may be complicated by hyperinflation of the remaining emphysematous lung, it is a simpler, shorter operation with a lower perioperative complication rate and is preferred for older, high risk patients and in those with previous unilateral thoracotomy or pleurodesis or marked asymmetry in function between the two lungs. Bilateral sequential lung transplantation may be preferable for younger, lower risk patients and those with significant bilateral disease and/or if an undersized donor is being considered.

Determining Side of Transplant

Fibrotic Lung Disease.   There is a surgical preference for transplanting the left lung due to greater ease of exposure and the longer left main bronchus, however in patients without previous surgery or chest tube insertion, either side may be transplanted. Many patients with fibrotic lung disease will have had diagnostic open lung biopsies performed and we preferentially transplant the side contralateral to previous thoracotomies.

Pulmonary Hypertension. In patients with Eisenmenger's physiology, the side of transplantation will depend on the cardiac anomaly. Atrial septal defects and small ventricular septal defects are corrected through a right sided thoracotomy, after which the right lung is replaced. Patients with a patent ductus arteriosus should have a left sided thoracotomy with left lung replacement. If a cardiovascular anomaly has been previously corrected via a thoracotomy, the side of transplantation will usually be contralateral to the previous incision.

In patients with primary pulmonary hypertension without a previous surgical procedure and without a patent foramen ovale, either lung may be transplanted. We currently perform preoperative differential ventilation-perfusion scans in these patients, but our experience is small and the importance of V/Q mismatching in determining side of transplantation is unknown.

Special Circumstances

While the above recommendations apply to most candidates, the introduction of transplantation to a wider variety of patients has required special considerations in their evaluation and preoperative management.

Pediatric Population

Although experience to date is small, children have successfully received heart-lung, double-lung, and single-lung transplants for a variety of disease entities. Heart disease that is otherwise inoperable has been the major indication, although children with fibrotic lung disease, CF, and bronchopulmonary dysplasia have also been transplanted.

Infants with disease of the pulmonary artery who appear to be developing intractable heart failure or who are failing to develop with maximal medical treatment should be considered. Children who have pulmonary hypertension are usually judged by the same criteria as adults: ability to climb stairs; to walk on the level; and to perform activities of daily living. There is no evidence that pulmonary hypertension is more or less relentless than in adults. Again, it is particularly important to consider the rate of decline of function rather than the absolute magnitude of hypertension in making a decision for candidacy.

Children who require mechanical ventilation for more than 1 or 2 days prior to surgery should be considered to have both lungs colonized with hospital-acquired organisms. These patients should probably receive heart-lung (or bilateral sequential lung) transplantation rather than a single-lung transplant regardless of the nature of the lung disease.

Cystic Fibrosis

Most transplantation centers now consider patients with CF as acceptable candidates for heart-lung or bilateral sequential transplantation. Indications for surgery in CF patients, including timing of listing for active candidacy, are identical to those chosen because of other disease entities. However we require that all prospective CF recipients have an ear-nose-throat evaluation prior to active candidacy. Most will require Caldwell-Luc antrostomies to provide access to the sinuses, followed by monthly antibiotic irrigation. This program of regular, prophylactic sinus flushing decreases the bacterial load of the upper respiratory tract and is continued posttransplant. We have found that this has been successful in decreasing the number of serious respiratory tract infections in this group.

There are some contraindications to transplantation that may be particularly common in the CF group. These are listed below.

Pleurodesis for Pneumothorax

There is still considerable danger in trying to remove a native lung with a great deal of pleural adhesions. Since pneumothorax in seriously ill CF patients is not uncommon, avoidance of surgical or chemical pleurodesis has become a therapeutic dilemma for those patients who may become future transplant candidates.

Respiratory Flora Resistant to all Available Antibiotics

Although the major portion of the bacterial burden of the respiratory tract is discarded with the native lungs, there will always be residual infection in the proximal trachea and paranasal sinuses. It will be necessary to suppress the growth of these organisms in the postoperative period, and thus panresistance is an absolute contraindication to transplantation.

Severe Cachexia Due to Poor Nutrition

This all-too-common condition in patients with severe CF may be amenable to treatment with enteral or parenteral hyperalimentation in the preoperative period.

Inability to Comply with the Strict Medical Regime
Necessary in the Postoperative Period

Although it seems incongruous, many older patients with CF have adopted definite ideas about the types of medication and treatments with which they will and will not comply. While this may seem courageous for a seriously ill patient in the final stages of their disease, this attitude has proven to be very destructive posttransplant when absolute compliance with a bewildering variety of drugs, dosages, and diagnostic procedures is necessary.

Smoking-Related Emphysema

Patients with smoking-related chronic obstructive airways disease must be vigorously investigated preoperatively to exclude other smoking related disease, specifically peripheral vascular disease, bronchogenic neoplasia, and upper airway malignancy. If patients are being considered for bilateral sequential lung or "domino" transplantation, coronary arteries are carefully assessed by arteriography.

Thus, in addition to the investigations outlined above, it is requested that all smokers fulfill the following criteria:

Abstinence from smoking for >2 years
Normal carotid duplex scan
Regular negative sputum cytology
Bronchoscopy with negative BAL cytology
Normal CT scan of chest
Normal ENT examination

(For double-lung/"domino" candidates only: normal coronary arteriogram with good left and right ventricular contractile function).

Acutely Ill Patients

Acutely ill patients or those requiring prolonged mechanical ventilation are generally not considered appropriate candidates for transplantation because of the propensity for infection, difficulty in assessment, and poor recovery. However increasing experience may allow such patients to be considered in exceptional cases.

Retransplantation Candidates

Posttransplant obliterative bronchiolitis affects up to 50% of heart-lung transplant candidates in some series, although the incidence and severity may be decreasing due to improvements in diagnosis and immunosuppressive therapy. In the absence of recurrent pulmonary infections, patients with severe disease may be considered for retransplantation (single lung transplant).

While the general principles of patient selection and assessment apply, these patients obviously have a history of previous cardiothoracic surgery and are at high risk for postoperative bleeding complications. Furthermore their immunosuppressed status increases the risks of infection, and chronic cyclosporine usage may have resulted in renal impairment. Preoperative evaluation should include coronary arteriograms to evaluate transplant coronary artery disease, careful renal assessment, and evaluation of anti-OKT3 antibody status if OKT3 immunosuppression was used at any time. This group of patients may have particular problems withdrawing from steroids, which may accelerate the primary disease and also precipitate acute rejection. Augmentation of azathioprine and cyclosporine to maximal tolerable levels is usually required.

Donor Evaluation and Management

Donor Evaluation

Heart-lung, single-lung, and bilateral sequential donors are evaluated and managed according to a single, standardized protocol. From the experience at Stanford it is estimated that only 10%-15% of cardiac donors meet the strict criteria for acceptable heart-lung or lung donors. Most lung donors are also acceptable heart donors. Only in exceptional circumstances has there been damage to the heart, or other pathology that would preclude cardiac donation, and yet permit lung donation. The general criteria for heart-lung or lung donor are outlined in Table 6. The donor should ideally be <45-years old, but donors as old as 55 should be considered. The donor should have no history of significant cardiac or pulmonary disease. Heavy smokers make poor lung donors, so only a minimal smoking history is acceptable. For the heart to be acceptable it must fulfill the usual cardiac donor criteria of having absence of prolonged hypotensive episodes, low dose inotrope support, and a normal electrocardiogram and echocardiogram.

The chest film should be absolutely clear. Most donors considered unsuitable are unacceptable on the basis of the chest film because of pulmonary infiltrates, neurogenic pulmonary edema, or evidence of pulmonary contusions. However, left lower lobe atelectasis is common in the intubated donor, can be reversed with transtracheal or bronchoscopic suctioning, and, in the absence of other evidence for pulmonary infection, does not constitute a contraindication to donation. Therefore, if the graft is otherwise suitable, the donor hospital is instructed that the donor team will perform bronchoscopy in the intensive care unit or the operating room to further assess the graft. Occasionally a donor will have a unilateral pulmonary contusion and the contralateral lung will still be acceptable for donation. Similarly, if a chest tube has been placed on one side but the other lung is intact with a clear film, then that lung would be acceptable for single-lung donation.

The arterial blood gases should also reflect excellent pulmonary function. As a guideline, the PaO_2 should be >100 mmHg on 40% FIO_2, and/or

---

Table 6
General Criteria for Heart-Lung or Lung Donors

1. Age <45 (but consider otherwise suitable donors up to age 55)
2. No history of cardiac or pulmonary disease
3. Minimal or negative smoking history
4. No prolonged hypotension or hypoxia
5. *Normal ECG and echocardiogram
6. Low dose inotrope support
7. Clear chest film
8. PaO_2 ≥100 mmHg on 0.4 F_iO_2 and/or
9. ≥400 mmHg on 1.0 F_iO_2
10. Peak inspiratory pressure <30 mmHg at ~15 cc/kg tidal volume
11. Negative pulmonary gram stain and KOH prep, or minimal bacterial contamination only

*Minor cardiac dysfunction may be acceptable for a single-lung donor

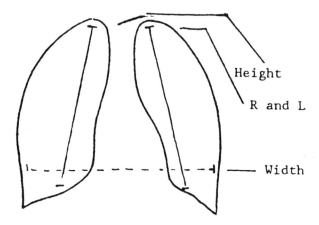

Figure 2. Chest measurements used to help assess donor-to-recipient size match.

the PaO_2 should be >400 mmHg on 100% FIO_2. To assure that the lung has normal compliance, the peak inspiratory pressures should be <30 mmHg at approximately 15 cc/kg tidal volume. Finally, an endotracheal tube aspirate should show no significant bacterial infection and total absence of fungal or yeast elements.

The donor coordinator needs the above information to make a decision regarding acceptability. Additional information includes donor height, weight, and chest measurements. The chest measurements are determined from the portable chest film. The width of the chest cavity is determined at the level of the diaphragm, and the heights of the right and left lungs are determined from the apices of the lungs to the tops of the diaphragms (Figure 2).

This information will be useful in determining the size match of the donor to recipient chest cavity. The donor hospital is instructed to place 5 liters of cold saline in ice to be used to help cool the graft at harvesting.

Donor Management

Management of the pulmonary donor is more difficult than management of a cardiac donor. First, the intravascular volume should be kept low to avoid pulmonary edema. We aim for a cental venous pressure (CVP) of 2–8 mmHg. Five percent albumin, or packed RBCs (cytomegalovirus negative, if possible), if necessary, can be used for volume. The mean arterial pressure should be maintained above 60 mmHg using dopamine and/or dobutamine (up to 10 mcg/kg per min) as with the management of most cardiac donors. If the patient is very vasodilated from neurogenic impairment, then the addition of neosynephrine to keep the mean arterial pressure over 60 mmHg is acceptable. If the urine output exceeds 200 mL/hr, then low doses of vasopressin are needed to facilitate intravascular volume management.

The management of the lungs requires frequent evaluation and careful attention to detail. Assiduous attempts should be made to keep the FIO_2 below 40%. PEEP may be added up to 5-cm H_2O. If the blood gases are deteriorating on these settings then the transplant team needs to be notified immediately of the deteriorating pulmonary status of the donor. Occasionally this will be due to secretions and the situation may be improved with frequent suctioning, turning, and intensive pulmonary care. While the transplant is being coordinated, the donor should have frequent chest films (every 6 hours) and blood gases every 1–2 hours, An oxygen saturation monitor should be placed on the patient. A stat gram stain and KOH prep of the pulmonary secretions should be sent. Also, the donor should be started on ceftazidime 1 gm intravenous (IV) q 6 hours, cefamandole 1 gm IV q 6 hours, and gentamicin 1 mg/kg IV q 8 hours. If there is uncertainty regarding the presence, occasionally donors have been intubated at the scene of an accident, or in the emergency room, with less than ideal endotracheal tubes. We prefer at least an 8.0 (ID) endotracheal tube with a low pressure, high volume cuff. One gram of methylprednisolone should be given IV before the donor goes to the operating room.

Donor Operation

Donor Anesthesia

In the operating room the anesthesiologist needs to insert two lines, if they have not already been placed. The donor needs a *right*-sided CVP line (because the innominate vein will be divided during the dissection) and a *left*-sided arterial line (because the innominate artery will also be divided). If a left radial, or brachial artery are not accessible, then the left carotid artery can be cannulated for arterial pressure monitoring. The FIO_2 should be kept $\leq$ 40% in the operating room, and preferably during transport from the intensive care unit to the operating room. We try to minimize the FIO_2 to decrease the risk of oxygen toxicity to the lungs. In the operating room the blood gases should be checked every 30 minutes. Any change from baseline should be reported to the donor surgeon. An oxygen saturation monitor should be placed. The timing of prostaglandin E1 infusion by the anesthesiologist is directed by the donor surgeon. The donor coordinator furnishes the anesthesiologist the cold cardioplegia solution with a pressure bag and also oversees setting up the cold pulmonary perfusion apparatus.

Heart-Lung Bloc Retrieval

The donor should be supine on the operating table with both arms tucked in at the sides, is prepped, and draped in the usual fashion. The sternotomy should be performed at the same time as the liver-kidney harvesting teams are starting, and the pericardium is opened in the midline and reflected laterally. The heart is closely inspected for evidence of contusions, regional wall motion abnormalities, and coronary artery disease. The heart is carefully palpated for any thrills, or other evidence of valvular pathology. Next, the pleural spaces are opened bilaterally and both lungs are inspected for pulmonary contusion, lacerations, consolidation, or pleural effusions. If the condition of the heart and lungs is acceptable, then the other teams involved should be asked to estimate when they will be ready for the heart-lung graft to be harvested. The condition of the graft and the anticipated time of removal should be phoned back to the recipient transplant team. It is important during the dissection to manipulate the lungs as little as possible because transplanted lungs are very susceptible to trauma.

Next, a near-complete pericardiectomy is performed, including resection of the phrenic nerves and the thymus. The innominate vein is divided in its midportion. The innominate artery may then be divided at this point. The superior vena cava (SVC) is encircled with two ties. The azygos vein is dissected free, doubly ligated, and divided. The inferior vena cava (IVC) is dissected circumferentially away from the diaphragm. The aortic arch and anterior pulmonary artery are dissected over to the level of the ligamentum arteriosum. A tape is passed around the aortic arch and it is retracted inferiorly and to the left. The trachea is exposed and dissected, starting approximately 3 inches above the carina. The dissection should be kept well away from the carina to preserve the peritracheal tissues, which contain the collateral blood supply from the coronary circulation. Care has to be taken to avoid entry into the esophagus (a previously passed nasogastric tube is helpful). The trachea is encircled with an umbilical tape. At this point there is usually a wait until the other donor teams have completed their dissection.

Approximately 15 minutes before the graft is ready to be harvested, 300 u/kg of heparin should be given IV. An initial infusion of prostaglandin E1 (25 ng/kg per min) is begun, and the dose is doubled every 2 minutes.

Prostaglandin E1 is a potent vasodilator, and as the dose is increased, systemic vasodilation and hypotension will occur. Ligation and division of the innominate artery at this point partly counteracts the tendency to hypotension. The cardioplegia line should be flushed, inserted, and secured. The pulmonary perfusion line (we have used either a 14 or 20 Fr left ventricular vent) is flushed and inserted into the main pulmonary artery (Figure 3).

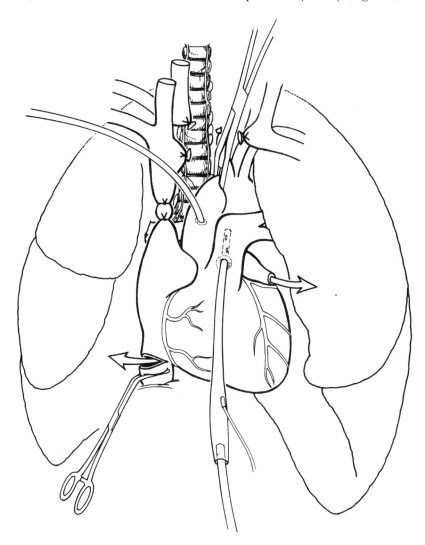

Figure 3. Harvesting of the heart-lung bloc. Cardioplegia is infused and vented through the IVC. Pulmonary infusion is vented through the left atrial appendage.

The pulmonary perfusion solution ("pulmonoplegia" in our vernacular) is a modified Euro Collins solution to each liter of which 8 mEq $MgSO_4$ and 65 cc of 50% dextrose have been added. Both are infused at 4°C through an in-line (5 micron) filter. When the other donor teams are ready for the graft to be removed, the prostaglandin E1 infusion is opened wide. As the systemic blood pressure drops, additional vasodilating drugs (chlorpromazine, phentolamine) may be given if requested by the renal donor team. After the infusions are given, the anesthesiologist withdraws the central line. The SVC is doubly ligated and divided. A spoon Potts clamp is placed on the IVC and the IVC is divided. The heart is allowed to beat empty for a few contractions and then the aortic cross-clamp is applied.

The cardioplegia infusion is then started in the ascending aorta and is vented via the coronary sinus through the opened IVC. The pulmonary artery infusion is begun simultaneously and the tip of the left atrial appendage is excised. The left atrial appendage should be opened widely to allow full egress of the pulmonary infusate (Figure 3). The pressure in the pulmonary artery during infusion should not exceed 20 mmHg. The pressure in the aorta should not exceed 100 mmHg during infusion. Perfusion cooling of the lungs is maintained at a rate of 15 cc/kg per min, for a total of 4 minutes. This should result in even "blanching" of both lungs. The anesthesiologist continues gentle ventilation by hand to facilitate even distribution of the perfusion fluid, but now uses compressed air instead of oxygen mixtures (this requires a compressed air source). Five liters of cold saline are topically applied to the heart and both lungs. When the cardioplegia solution is completely infused, the line is removed from the ascending aorta. When the pulmonary perfusion solution has been infused, the line is removed from the pulmonary artery.

The aorta is transected at the level of the innominate artery. The anesthesiologist is instructed to moderately inflate the lungs and slowly withdraw the endotracheal tube. Two large Kocher clamps are applied to the high trachea when the endotracheal tube has been retracted to the level of the vocal cords. In this way the lung grafts will be harvested with the lungs inflated with air. The trachea is divided between the clamps (Figure 4). Alternatively, a stapler may be used at this point.

The inferior trachea and the aorta are retracted to the patient's left. The cautery is used to dissect behind the trachea being careful to avoid opening the esophagus. The blood supply to the trachea runs along the side of the trachea at the 3 and 9 o'clock positions. As much peritracheal tissue as possible should be preserved with the graft. The dissection continues down to the level of the azygos vein, which is divided (if it was not already divided). The right pulmonary ligament is divided with cautery. The right lung is carefully retracted to the left and the dissection continues along the posterior mediastinum. The majority of the posterior mediastinum can be dissected at this stage. Care has to be taken not to injure the right pulmonary artery or the right bronchus. When the level of the ligamentum arteriosum is reached on the left, then the right lung should be replaced into the right chest. The surgeon retracts the left lung superiorly and to the right. The assistant divides the left pulmonary ligament and completes the

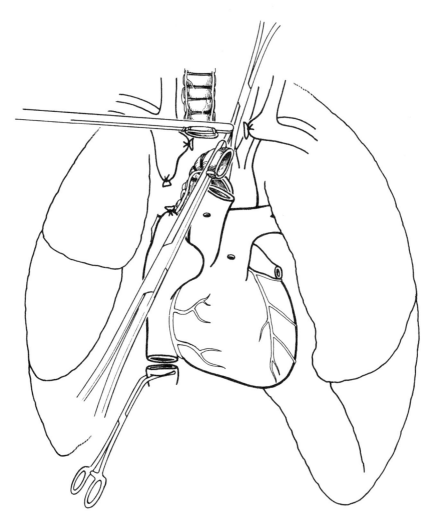

Figure 4. The infusion catheters have been removed. The aorta is divided and then the trachea. The graft is rotated inferiorly and to the left and dissection begins in the posterior mediastinum on the right side.

posterior mediastinal dissection using the cautery. The heart-lung bloc is then removed to the back table.

The trachea is stapled (if this has not already been done) just below the clamp using a TA 55 stapling device. The heart-lung graft is thoroughly rinsed with several liters of cold saline. It is placed into a bowel bag with approximately 1 liter of Physiosol solution. A moistened laparotomy pad is placed on each lung (be careful of the sponge count at the recipient's operation!) to help immerse the lungs. The bowel bag is tied and placed into a second bowel bag, which contains approximately 1/2 liter of Physiosol. This bag is placed into a plastic container that is then sealed. The plastic container is placed into the ice chest and thoroughly surrounded with ice. The graft is ready for transport.

Special Harvesting Techniques

Domino Transplant

Several technical points deserve mention for harvesting in special circumstances. First, if the heart-lung graft is being used for a domino transplant (a recipient whose own heart will be excised and used for another transplant), then dissection of the SVC needs to be extended in both donor and heart-lung recipient. In a domino transplant procedure we now perform a direct anastomosis of the donor SVC to that of the recipient. This anastomosis must be done high above the sinoatrial node to avoid sinus node dysfunction in the recipient of the heart from the domino transplant. Therefore, the donor SVC should be divided above the junction with the azygos vein.

Separation of Heart from Heart-Lung Bloc

When the heart will be used separately for heart transplantation, it should be removed after the cardioplegia and pulmonary perfusion solutions have been infused. If only a left lung graft will be used, then the left atrium is divided midway between the coronary sinus and left pulmonary veins. The right pulmonary veins can be divided at the level of the pericardium. The aorta and pulmonary artery are divided in the usual fashion. The critical part of this extraction involves division of the left atrium so as to leave adequate cuffs for both the heart and the lung transplant teams.

For a right lung transplant, or bilateral lung transplant, the interatrial groove on the right-side has to be dissected. This dissection will leave adequate atrial cuff for the lung transplants and sufficient atrial tissue for the heart transplant. Ideally this dissection should be performed while the other donor teams are completing their dissection, and while the heart is full and beating. Approximately 1–3 cm can be dissected in the right interatrial groove. If for some reason this dissection has not been performed before removal of the graft(s), it can be carried out after the harvesting, utilizing traction on the IVC and SVC to facilitate exposure of the groove.

Double-Lung Transplant (Bilateral Sequential)

If the recipient will receive both lungs as a bilateral sequential lung transplant, then the heart should be excised after dissection in the interatrial groove on the right, and division of the mid-left atrium, as described above. In addition, the pulmonary artery needs to be divided through its bifurcation and the airway is divided at the level of the carina. This will ensure sufficient pulmonary artery and bronchus for each side of the bilateral sequential lung transplant.

Selected References

1. Baldwin JC, Frist WH, Starkey TD, et al. Distant graft procurement for combined heart and lung transplantation using pulmonary artery flush and simple topical hypothermia for graft preservation. Ann Thorac Surg 1987;43:670–673.
2. Baumgartner WA, Traill TA, Cameron DE, et al. Unique aspects of heart and lung transplantation exhibited in the "domino donor" operation. JAMA 1989; 261:3121–3125.
3. Bolman RM, Shumay SJ, Estrin J, et al. Lung and heart-lung transplantation. Evolution and new applications. Ann Surg 1991;214:456–470.
4. Carere R, Patterson GA, Liu P, et al. Right and left ventricular performance following single and double lung transplantation. J Thorac Cardiovasc Surg 1991;102:115–122.
5. Egan TM, Kaiser LR, Cooper JD. Lung transplantation. Curr Prob Surg 1989;26: 673–752.
6. Harjula A, Baldwin JC, Starnes VA, et al. Proper donor selection for heart-lung transplantation. J Thorac Cardiovasc Surg 1987;94:874–880.
7. Harjula A, Baldwin JC, Stinson EB, et al. Clinical heart-lung preservation with prostaglandin E-1. Transplant Proc 1987;14:4101–4102.
8. Hakim M, Higenbottam T, Bethune D, et al. Selection and procurement of combined heart and lung grafts for transplantation. J Thorac Cardiovasc Surg 1988;95:474–479.
9. Hakim M, Higenbottam T, English TAH, et al. Distant procurement and preservation of heart-lung homografts. Tranplant Proc 1987;5:3535–3536.

10. Jamieson SW, Stinson EB, Oyer PE, et al. Operative technique for heart-lung transplantation: The Stanford experience. J Appl Cardiology 1987;2:71–89.
11. Kawaguchi A, Ganddjbakhch I, Pavie A, et al. Heart and unilateral lung transplantation in patients with end-stage cardiopulmonary disease and previous thoracic operations. J Thorac Cardiovasc Surg 1989;98:343–349.
12. Kramer MR, Tiroke A, Marshall SE, et al. The clinical significance of hyperbilirubinemia in patients with pulmonary hypertension under-going heart-lung transplant. J Heart Transplant 1990;9:79.
13. Harjula A, Baldwin JC, Starnes VA, et al. Proper donor selection for heart-lung transplantation. J Thorac Cardiovasc Surg 1987;94:874–880.
14. Low DE, Tmlock EP, Kaiser LR, et al. Morbidity, mortality, and early results of single versus bilateral lung transplantation for emphysema. J Thorac Cardiovasc Surg 1992;103:1119–1126.
15. Marshall SE, Kramer MR, Lewiston NJ, et al. Selection and evaluation of recipients for heart-lung and lung transplantation. Chest 1990;98:1488–1494.
16. McCarthy PM, Starnes VA, Theodore J, et al. Improved survival after heart-lung transplantation. J Thorac Cardiovasc Surg 1990;99:54–60.
17. Reitz BA. Adapted indications for lung transplantation. Discussion report. J Heart Lung Transplant 1992;14:5286–5296.
18. Reitz BA, Wallwork JL, Hunt SA, et al. Heart-lung transplantation: Successful therapy for patients with pulmonary vascular disease. N Engl J Med 1982;306:557–564.
19. Shennib H, Noirclerc M, Ernst P, et al. Cystic fibrosis transplant study group. Double-lung transplantation for cystic fibrosis. Ann Thorac Surg 1992;54:27–32.
20. Shumway SJ, Burdine J, Bolman RM III. Combined harvest of heart and lungs. Techniques and results. Transplant Proc 1991;23:1236–1238.
21. Todd TR, Goldberg M, Koshal A, et al. Separate extraction of cardiac and pulmonary grafts from a single organ donor. Ann Thorac Surg 1988;46:356–359.
22. Toronto Lung Transplant Group. Unilateral lung transplantation for pulmonary fibrosis. N Engl J Med 1986;314:1140–1145.
23. Yacoub MH, Banner NR, Chaghani A, et al. Heart-lung transplantation for cystic fibrosis and subsequent domino heart transplantation. J Heart Transplant 1990;9:459–467.
24. Zenati M, Dowling RD, Armitage JM, et al. Organ procurement for pulmonary transplantation. Ann Thorac Surg 1989;48:882–886.

Chapter 10

Preoperative Evaluation, Anesthetic Management, Operative Techniques, and Postoperative Routines for Heart-Lung and Lung Transplantation

Patrick M. McCarthy, M.D., George E. Sarris, M.D., Lawrence C. Siegel, M.D., Edward B. Stinson, M.D.

Heart-lung and lung transplantation is generally more demanding than routine heart transplantation for the surgeons, nurses, anesthesiologists, pulmonologists, and especially the patients. Preoperatively, these patients must be carefully evaluated. Some may have deteriorated since their last visit and become "too sick" to undergo transplant. The operations, anesthetic management, and postoperative care can be difficult and mistakes in management are not well tolerated.

Preoperative Evaluation

As outlined in Chapter 3, the initial telephone conversation is used to reevaluate the patient's physical status. For heart-lung transplant patients, the onset of rising bilirubin, ascites, peripheral edema, weight gain, and other evidence of worsening right-heart failure indicates that the patient should be "deactivated" until increasing medical management can improve his/her pretransplant condition. As with all transplant operations, a recent fever, or active infection is usually a contraindication to transplantation. An exception is made for patients with cystic fibrosis, or bronchiectasis, who may have infection confined just to the lung. For these patients it may be acceptable to proceed with transplantation being careful to minimize contamination at the operation.

From: Smith JA, McCarthy PM, Sarris GE, Stinson EB, Reitz BA (eds.): The Stanford Manual of Cardiopulmonary Transplantation. Futura Publishing Co., Inc., Armonk, NY, 1996.

Transportation and admission to the hospital are arranged the same as for heart transplantation. The pretransplant medications are also essentially the same. Cyclosporine is not given preoperatively. Azathioprine (4 mg/kg intravenously [IV]) is given, however. Fresh frozen plasma and vitamin K are especially important for those with liver dysfunction. The appropriate consents are obtained and the patient is sent to the operating room, usually about the same time the donor team has arrived at the other hospital.

Anesthetic Management of the Heart-Lung Transplant Recipient

Preoperative Anesthetic Evaluation

The standard preanesthetic evaluation is supplemented with considerations particular to these patients. The progression of disease is usually well documented in these chronically ill patients. A history of recent exacerbation of symptoms should be sought and cardiac catheterization data should be interpreted in light of interval changes.

The severity of pulmonary hypertension and the responsiveness to specific vasodilators during catheterization should be reviewed. Intracardiac shunting may be present in patients with pulmonary hypertension, and a history of embolic episodes should be sought. Patients with severe pulmonary hypertension have large pulmonary arteries. Vocal cord dysfunction may occur when the left recurrent laryngeal nerve is stretched by an enlarged pulmonary artery. These patients are at increased risk for pulmonary aspiration. Evidence of renal and hepatic dysfunction should be sought by history, physical examination, and laboratory studies.

Hypokalemia should not be treated because the heart-lung graft is preserved with potassium and implantation will reverse hypokalemia. The medication schedule should be verified with particular attention to the recent use of vasodilators, inotropes, diuretics, antidysrhythmics, anticoagulants, immunosuppressive agents, and noncardiovascular medications.

Although appropriately anxious, patients awaiting heart-lung transplantation are generally well informed about the planned perioperative course. These patients respond well to the reassurance of the preoperative visit and pharmacologic premedication is usually not necessary.

Oxygen therapy should commence prior to transport of the patient to the operating room.

Anesthetic Equipment and Monitoring

Upon arrival in the operating room, the patient should be placed on the operating table and oxygen and noninvasive monitors should be applied. A patient who is dyspneic in the supine position may be treated by raising the back of the operating table.

Noninvasive monitors include pulse oximetry, five-lead electrocardiography with ST segment analysis (leads should be covered with tape to ensure that electrical contact is not degraded by prep solution or blood), automated blood pressure measurement, and precordial stethoscope.

Infection is a much feared complication in the immunosuppressed transplant patient; thus, aseptic technique is important. Airway equipment is presterilized. A disposable circuit system and bacterial filters are used. Aseptic technique is used in inserting and securing all vascular catheters.

Patients with intracardiac defects are at increased risk for cerebral embolic events. Care must be taken to remove all air bubbles from intravascular lines.

Two 14- or 16-gauge IV catheters are inserted because bleeding is often a major problem after termination of cardiopulmonary bypass. Midazolam (0.5 mg) or fentanyl (50 ug) may be titrated IV to assure patient comfort. A 20-gauge catheter is placed percutaneously in a radial artery. A triple lumen central venous catheter or an 8.5 Fr introducer is usually inserted prior to the induction of anesthesia. If the patient is very dyspneic in the supine position, or if the initial time estimate for the arrival of the graft is substantially in error, it may be advantageous to insert the central venous catheter following anesthetic induction. An introducer permits the rapid insertion of a pulmonary artery catheter when necessary. The left internal jugular vein is the preferred site of cannulation, leaving the right internal jugular unscarred for repeated endomyocardial biopsies of the transplanted heart.

The anesthesia machine should be equipped with a supply of air to permit control of the F_iO_2.

Anesthetic Induction and Maintenance

Anesthesia is not induced until the team harvesting the graft reports that it appears to be normal to direct inspection. The patient is denitrogenated with $F_iO_2 = 1.0$. Continuous airway gas analysis should be used.

Cricoid pressure must be used when the patient is at risk for pulmonary aspiration of gastric contents because of the unscheduled nature of the surgery, and vocal cord dysfunction associated with stretch injury of the recurrent laryngeal nerve.

A major goal of anesthetic induction is the avoidance of further increases in pulmonary vascular resistance (PVR). Avoid respiratory acidosis. Avoid hypoxia. Avoid extremes of lung volume. Adequate depth of anesthesia is necessary. Nitrous oxide should be avoided because it can exacerbate high PVR.

When hemodynamically tolerated, fentanyl, 30 ug/kg, is useful in blunting the pulmonary vascular responsiveness to endotracheal intubation. Etomidate (0.1–0.2 mg/kg) may be used when hypotension limits the administration of narcotics. Vecuronium (0.15 mg/kg), pancuronium (0.1 mg/kg), or a combination of these agents should be administered early to permit rapid control of the airway. Midazolam and scopolamine produce amnesia. Nitrous oxide is not used because it exacerbates pulmonary hypertension, reduces F_iO_2, and expands intravascular air bubbles.

The patient should be ventilated by mask and cricoid pressure released only after the airway has been secured with a cuffed endotracheal tube. Excessive pressure of the endotracheal tube cuff upon the trachea should be avoided. An endotracheal tube with an internal diameter of 8.0 mm will facilitate fiberoptic bronchoscopy postoperatively.

Antibiotics are administered and a urinary catheter with a thermistor is inserted. Additional monitors including a nasopharyngeal temperature probe and an esophageal stethoscope are placed. Insertion of an oral-gastric tube will facilitate location of the esophagus intraoperatively. If there is a delay in the anticipated arrival of the graft, the recipient should be covered and kept warm and the skin prep should be delayed.

Typical total anesthetic doses for the entire intraoperative course:

1. Fentanyl 50 ug/kg or sufentanil 10–15 ug/kg
2. Midazolam 0.2 mg/kg
3. Vecuronium 0.3 mg/kg or pancuronium 0.2 mg/kg
4. Scopolamine 0.07 mg/kg

Termination of Cardiopulmonary Bypass

After the tracheal anastomosis is completed, the lung is ventilated with $F_iO_2 = 0.21$ at 5 breaths/minute and a tidal volume of 6 mL/kg. When the bladder temperature reaches 36° C, ventilation is increased to a rate of 10 breaths/minute and a tidal volume of 12 mL/kg. The tidal volume should be adjusted to eliminate atelectasis and to achieve a peak inflation pressure of 25–30 cm H_2O with the chest open. The F_iO_2 is increased to 0.4 and may be altered in response to pulse oximetry and blood gas data. F_iO_2 is limited in the hope of curtailing free radical injury. Positive end expiratory pressure (PEEP) may be used to enhance oxygenation. PEEP is adjusted with an appreciation of the effect of lung volume on PVR. Hypoxemia is unacceptable.

Junctional rhythm is common in the denervated transplanted heart. Isoproterenol 10–75 ng/kg per min is used to achieve a heart rate of 100–120 beats/minute. When sinus rhythm is achieved, it is common to observe two P waves. As with an orthotopic heart transplant, the residual atrial tissue produces nonconducting P waves. Responses mediated by vagal tone will be observed in the rate of the original atrial tissue and have no clinical importance beyond the ease with which the electrocardiogram is interpreted. Atropine and neostigmine do not affect heart rate. Hypertension does not produce reflex bradycardia. The graft atrium produces normally conducted P waves. The graft conductive tissue contains adrenergic receptors and responds in a directionally appropriate manner to norepinephrine, epinephrine, and isoproterenol.

The cardiac output of the denervated heart is quite sensitive to preload; thus, IV fluid and vasodilators must be given with particular care. Sodium nitroprusside is used for afterload reduction. Prostaglandin E1 and nitroglycerin may also be used as needed for pulmonary vasodilation. Inotropic support with dopamine and epinephrine may be necessary, especially if pulmonary hypertension and right ventricular failure occur.

Post-bypass bleeding is a common problem exacerbated by preoperative use of anticoagulants, depressed synthetic function of the liver, trauma of cardiopulmonary bypass, and previous chest operation.

Coagulation therapy includes protamine, epsilon amino-caproic acid, and red blood cells and DDAVP. Blood products are avoided if possible. Severe bleeding prompts further therapy: platelets, fresh frozen plasma, and cryoprecipitate. Factor IX concentrate may be used if severe coagulopathy persists, but should be avoided as it carries a substantial risk for hepatitis. Recently, aprotinin has been utilized in selected patients, and appears to be of benefit.

For further immunosuppression, methylprednisolone 500 mg is given after bypass is terminated and protamine is given. There may be little urine production, especially if the patient received high dose diuretics preoperatively. Cyclosporine may exacerbate renal dysfunction and is not used preoperatively. Diuresis may be induced with mannitol and furosemide. Pulmonary edema may be a problem given the lack of lymphatic drainage. Diuresis, restriction of IV fluids, and utilization of dopamine (rather than volume) to support blood pressure is important.

Heart-Lung Transplant Operative Technique

Routine

The procedure is performed through a median sternotomy. The patient is cannulated for cardiopulmonary bypass using the usual technique for heart transplant with an arterial cannula in the ascending aorta and two caval cannulas (Figure 1). Cardiopulmonary bypass is established and the patient is cooled to 28° C. The heart is excised in the typical fashion as for heart transplantation starting with a right atrial incision, then transecting the aorta, pulmonary artery, and finally left atrium (Figure 2).

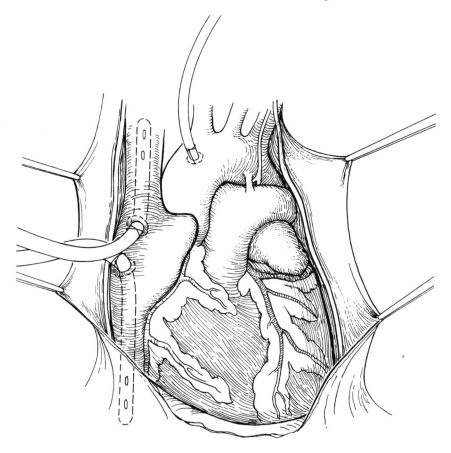

Figure 1. Cannulation for heart-lung transplant.

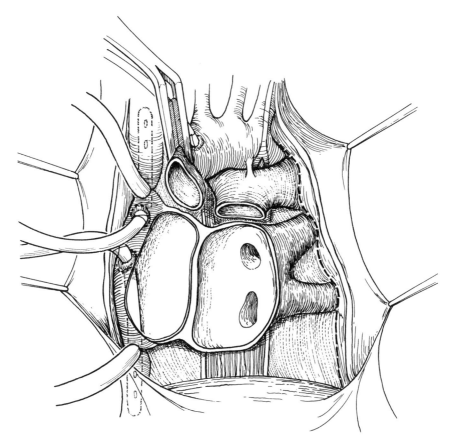

Figure 2. The heart is excised. The dotted line marks the planned pericardial division below the phrenic nerve.

The left pleural space is opened and the anterior pericardium is partially resected leaving a cuff approximately 3 cm anterior to the left phrenic nerve. The left atrium is divided between the left and right pulmonary veins posteriorly (Figure 3). The pericardium is then opened adjacent to the left pulmonary veins and this incision is extended superiorly and inferiorly below the phrenic nerve. This technique should leave a pedicle with the phrenic nerve totally intact and surrounded by approximately 1–2 cm posteriorly and 3 cm anteriorly. The incision has to be extended superiorly and inferiorly to the diaphragm to allow easy insertion of the left lung graft underneath the phrenic pedicle (Figure 4).

The pulmonary artery is divided in the midportion. The area of the lig-

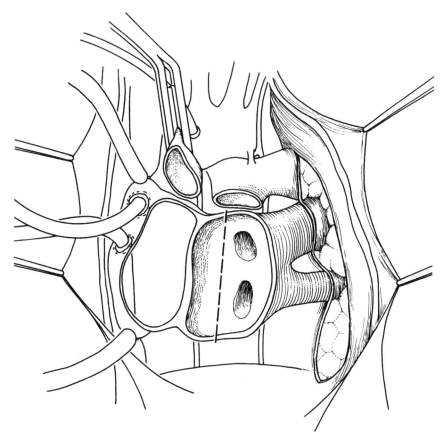

Figure 3. The posterior left atrial wall is divided. Do not open the pericardium in the posterior mediastinum behind this.

amentum arteriosum is identified and a small button (about 2 cm) of pulmonary artery is preserved in order to protect the left recurrent laryngeal nerve (Figure 5). The left pulmonary veins and left pulmonary artery are mobilized from the surrounding corrective tissue and retracted laterally (underneath the phrenic pedicle) into the left pleural space. Cautery is used to dissect out the left bronchus, which is transected with a TA 55 stapler with 4.8-mm staples (Figure 6). The inferior pulmonary ligament is divided carefully. The left lung is removed (Figure 7). Collateral vessels may be encountered, which can lead to troublesome bleeding, and must be diligently controlled. During the manipulation and dissection of septic lung tissue (e.g., cystic fibrosis) shed blood should be aspirated to wall suction and discarded, not returned to the cardiotomy reservoir. Otherwise, the

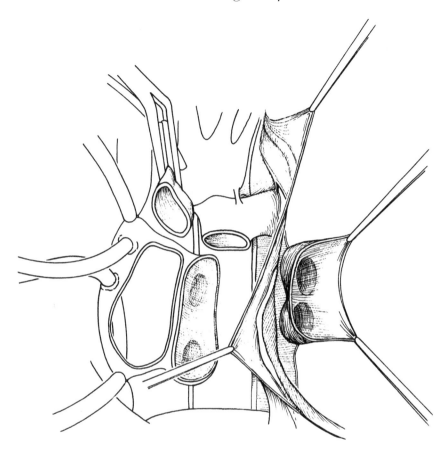

Figure 4. The left pulmonary veins can be retracted laterally underneath the phrenic pedicle.

products of bacterial contamination may profoundly depress systemic vasomotor tone and lead to a shock-like state.

The posterior pericardium should be left intact as much as possible to avoid hemorrhage from the posterior mediastinum. The right pleural space is entered and the right anterior pericardium is then excised (Figure 8). The right pulmonary vein and right pulmonary artery are mobilized. Care has to be taken on the right side when dividing the pericardium adjacent to the pulmonary veins because the right phrenic nerve may be very close. The right inferior pulmonary ligament is divided, the bronchus is mobilized, and the right bronchus is divided with a TA 55 stapler. The right lung is then removed (Figure 9). The carina of the trachea is mobilized anteriorly and posteriorly but only for a distance of approximately 1 cm. This

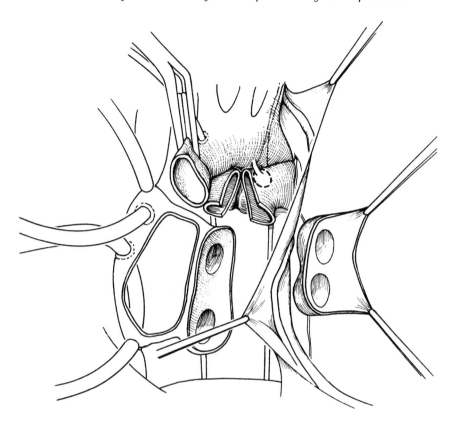

Figure 5. The recurrent laryngeal nerve is preserved by leaving a portion of pulmonary artery around the ductal remnant.

maneuver is facilitated by placing traction on each of the stapled main bronchi in a claudal direction. The lateral peritracheal tissues are preserved because the blood supply runs along the lateral margin of the trachea. The inferior portion of the carina is transsected (Figure 10). There is usually brisk bleeding from the cut edges that should be controlled with cautery.

With the heart and both lungs removed (Figure 11), the mean arterial perfusion pressure should be increased to approximately 90 mmHg. Careful hemostasis must be obtained in the posterior mediastinum and along the area where the pulmonary ligaments were divided. Any intrapleural adhesions are also a troublesome source of bleeding and these sites should be carefully inspected.

The right lung of the heart-lung graft is passed underneath the right atrium and right phrenic nerve pedicle (Figure 12). The left lung is then

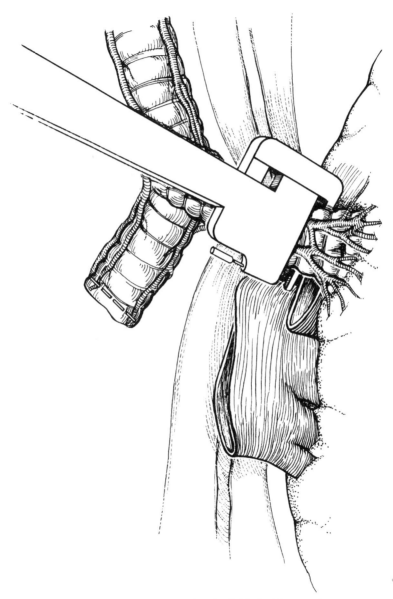

Figure 6. The left bronchus is divided with a stapler.

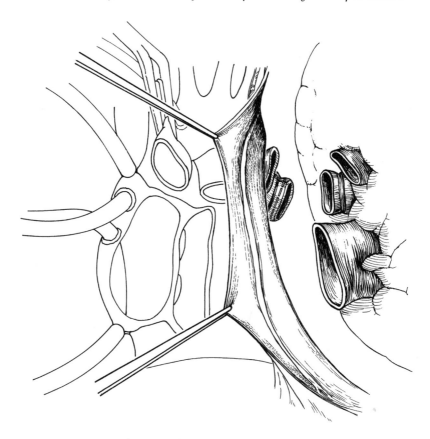

Figure 7. Completed dissection of the left lung.

passed underneath the left phrenic pedicle. Care must be taken to verify proper location of all lobes of the lung without any torsion or kinking. Manipulation of the lungs should be kept to a minimum to avoid injury. The tracheal anastomosis is sutured end-to-end with running or interrupted 3–0 polypropolene (Figure 13). The sutures are placed 1–2 mm apart and 1–2 mm from the cut edge of the trachea. We do not "telescope" the donor into recipient trachea, or wrap the anastomosis with omentum. The anterior peritracheal tissues (donor to recipient) are approximated with running 4–0 polypropolene. This suture line covers and seals the anastomosis and separates it from the aortic anastomosis. Ventilation is started with air, tidal volume 6 mL/kg and 5 breaths/minute.

The donor right atrium is opened from the inferior vena cava (IVC) to the base of the right atrial appendage as for a routine heart transplant. The

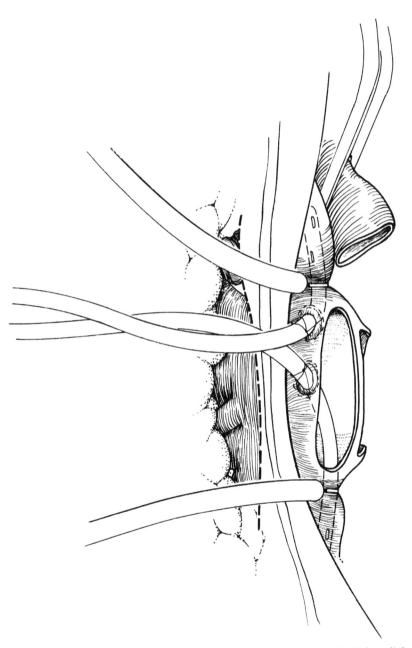

Figure 8. A pedicle for the right phrenic nerve is prepared similar to the left pedicle.

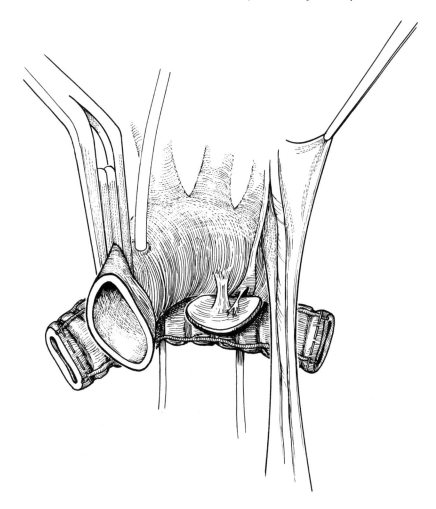

Figure 9. The right pulmonary artery and veins have been dissected out and the bronchus stapled and transected.

right atrial anastomosis is performed with running 3–0 polypropolene suture (Figure 14). The aortic anastomosis is then performed with running 4–0 polypropolene suture (Figure 15). Air is evacuated from the heart and the aortic cross-clamp is removed. The vent sites on the left atrial appendage and pulmonary artery are closed. The pericardium of donor and recipient is loosely approximated to form a "cradle" for the heart.

Atrial and ventricular pacing wires are placed. The F_iO_2 is increased to 0.4 and full ventilation is begun (10–15 mL/kg; 10 breaths/minute). The

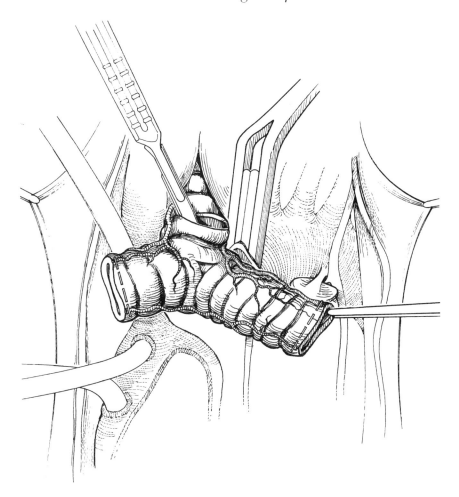

Figure 10. The trachea is divided just above the carina. The lateral peritracheal blood supply is illustrated. The associated lymph nodes and connective tissue that must also be preserved are not shown.

patient is weaned from cardiopulmonary bypass and decannulated in the usual fashion (Figure 16). Methylprednisolone 500 mg is given IV after protamine administration. The oxygen saturation should be closely monitored after weaning the patient from cardiopulmonary bypass. PEEP (usually 5 cm H_2O) should be added to improve oxygenation. The peak inspiratory pressure ideally should be kept < 30 cm H_2O. Problems with graft preservation may be manifested early by hypoxemia with increasing oxygen requirements. The mediastinum and both pleural cavities are drained and

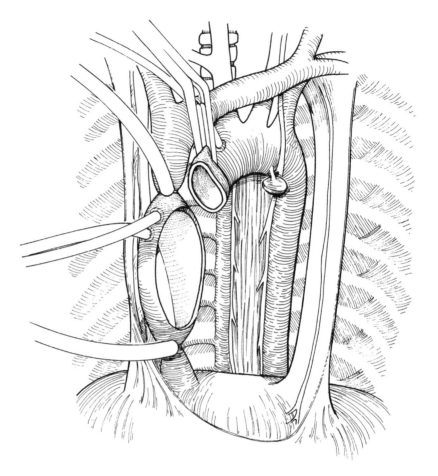

Figure 11. The recipient organs have been excised. The vagus nerves are seen along-side the esophagus for illustrative purposes. The posterior pericardium should be left in place to avoid bleeding from the posterior mediastinum.

the chest is closed, being careful to secure excellent approximation of the sternum.

A recent modification has been to perform heart-lung transplantation with caval anastomoses in a similar way to cardiac transplantation (Chapter 3). Improved right atrial shape results from this technique. In addition, we have placed the right and left lung hila in front of both phrenic nerve pedicles. This has not resulted in any damage to the phrenic nerves and makes it easier to rotate the lung out of the chest to look for posterior mediastinal bleeding after the patient is off bypass.

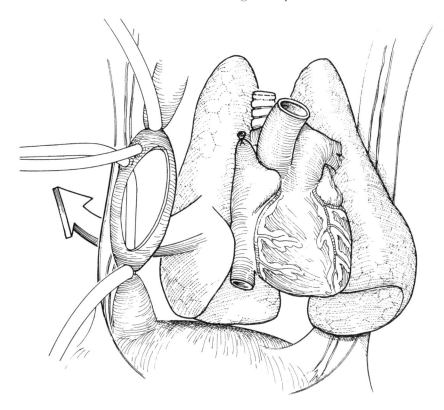

Figure 12. The heart-lung graft is placed by passing the right lung underneath the right atrium and right phrenic nerve pedicle.

Domino Heart-Lung Transplant

For this group of heart-lung recipients (typically with cystic fibrosis or alpha-1-antitrypsin deficiency) function of the heart is determined to be acceptable by preoperative tests and intraoperative inspection. Because such hearts frequently have moderate right ventricular hypertrophy from elevated PVR they are excellent donor hearts for patients who have modest elevations of PVR.

Because of increasing experience with bilateral sequential lung transplantation, however, "domino" heart transplantation is being performed less frequently. The heart-lung recipient and heart transplant recipient are anesthetized simultaneously in adjoining operating rooms. Two transplant surgical teams are necessary.

The heart-lung recipient is cannulated differently than usual, the vena

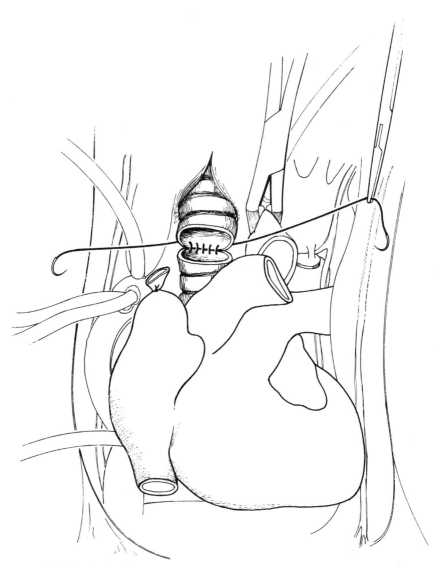

Figure 13. The tracheal anastomosis is performed with running 3–0 polypropolene. Not illustrated is the approximation of donor to recipient peritracheal tissue after the anastomosis has been completed.

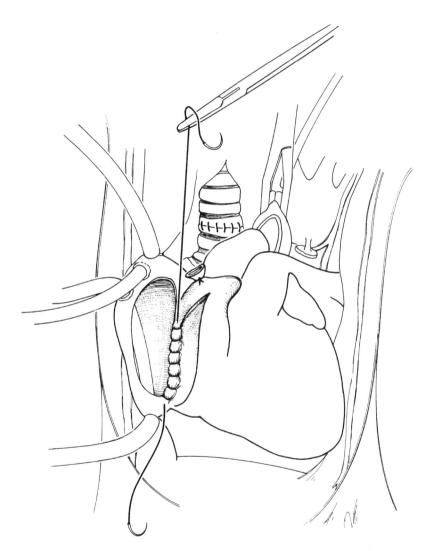

Figure 14. The right atrial anastomosis is performed as for a routine heart transplant.

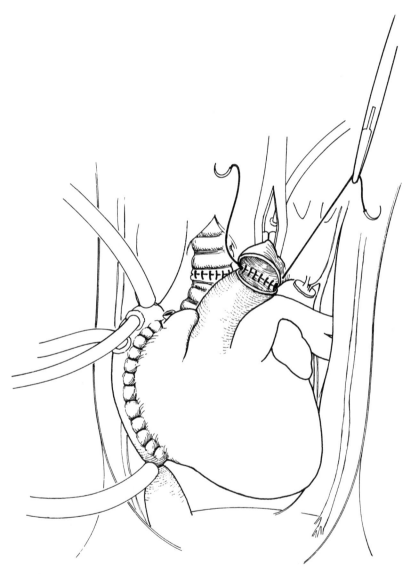

Figure 15. The aortic anastomosis is performed with running 4–0 polypropolene.

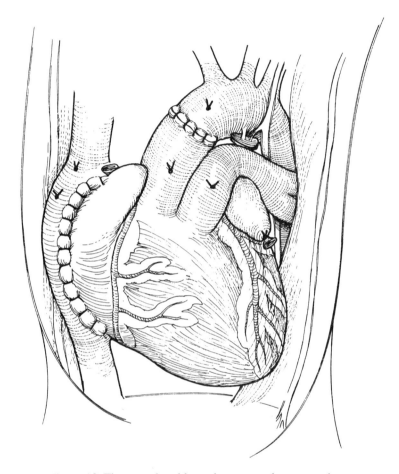

Figure 16. The completed heart-lung transplant operation.

cavae being cannulated directly. The superior vena cava (SVC) cannula should be very high. The heart is excised from the heart-lung recipient after cardioplegia is administered. The SVC is divided approximately 3 cm above the sinoatrial node. The IVC, aorta, pulmonary veins, and pulmonary artery are divided in the usual fashion for donor cardiectomy (see Chapter 2) except that a small cuff of pulmonary artery is preserved around the ligamentum arteriosum (Figure 5). The heart is placed in a basin of cold saline and taken to the adjacent operating room. It is implanted by the usual techniques for heart transplantation using separate SVC and IVC anastomoses (Chapter 3).

The heart-lung graft is placed in the recipient's chest in the usual fashion. After the tracheal anastomosis, the IVC and SVC are anastomosed directly end-to-end, unlike the usual right atrial anastomosis. The aortic anastomosis and remainder of the operation are routine.

Cystic Fibrosis Patients

Patients with cystic fibrosis have chronic lung infection and may be transplanted even though they have a fever related to their pulmonary disease (Figure 17). Extracting the lungs from the pleural spaces may be extremely difficult due to pleural adhesions. Postoperative bleeding may be a problem in these patients. Epsilon amino-caproic acid, tranexamic acid, or aproptinin is used, and procoagulants and fibrin glue may be necessary. Occasionally, a bilateral transverse thoracosternotomy ("clamshell") incision is used to improve visualization of the pleural spaces and control of bleeding from adhesions. We have found the Argon-beam coagulator to be quite useful in controlling bleeding from the diffusely oozing pleural surface after lysis of extensive adhesions.

In addition, the trachea and endotracheal tube may be contaminated from the pulmonary infection. Therefore, after the lungs have been removed, while the bronchi are still stapled we irrigate with dilute betadine through the endotracheal tube. This irrigant is then aspirated and the endotracheal tube is replaced with a new endotracheal tube. Care is taken to suction the secretions when the trachea is divided and the contaminated suckers are removed from the sterile field. The remainder of the operation is routine.

Anesthetic Management of the Single-Lung Transplant Recipient

Preoperative Anesthetic Evaluation

The preanesthetic evaluation is similar to the pre-heart-lung transplant considerations covered earlier in this chapter. In addition, evidence of right ventricular dysfunction should be sought. Right ventricular ejection fraction has usually been evaluated with radionuclide ventriculography. The severity of pulmonary hypertension and the responsiveness to specific vasodilators during catheterization should be reviewed. Review of the ventilation-perfusion scan will provide some insight into the changes expected when the patient is placed in the lateral position and when single lung ventilation is instituted. For those patients with pulmonary fibrosis the extent of the restrictive lung disease and diffusion abnormality can be assessed from the pulmonary function tests.

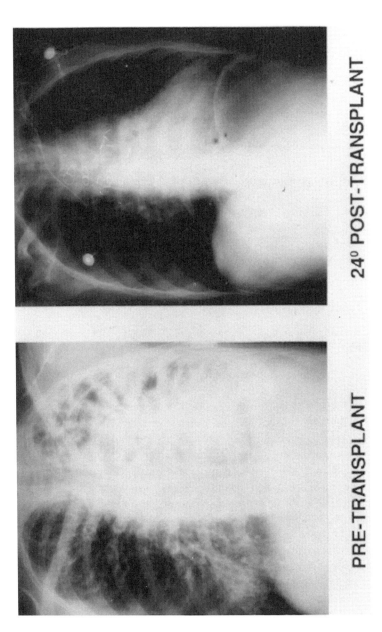

PRE-TRANSPLANT

24⁰ POST-TRANSPLANT

Figure 17. A cystic fibrosis patient with fever upon admission for heart-lung transplant. Twenty-four hours after removal of her infected lung tissue she was extubated with excellent graft function, and no infectious complications developed.

Intracardiac shunting and vocal cord dysfunction may be a problem as mentioned earlier.

Anesthetic Equipment and Monitoring

The equipment and monitoring are the same as for heart-lung transplant except that an 8.5 Fr introducer and a thermodilution pulmonary artery catheter are inserted prior to the induction of anesthesia. The catheter should be advanced into the main pulmonary artery. The right internal jugular vein may be used for cannulation.

Induction of Anesthesia and Anesthetic Agents

The only difference from heart-lung transplant is that a disposable PVC double lumen endobronchial tube is inserted in the left mainstem bronchus. Verification of tube position by auscultation may be quite difficult due to the severity of the lung disease. Fiberoptic bronchoscopy is used to verify proper tube placement. Proper positioning of the bronchial cuff in the proximal left mainstem bronchus does not interfere with surgical access to the bronchus.

Maintenance of Anesthesia

Isoflurane may be used if hypoxemia and right heart failure do not occur. Additional narcotics may be used if gas exchange or right heart function are a problem. The position of the double lumen endobronchial tube should be verified after the patient is moved to the lateral position. One lung ventilation is used to facilitate surgical access to the pulmonary artery and bronchus. Oxygenation must be watched closely; pulse oximetry is continuously monitored and arterial blood gases are sampled frequently. Transcutaneous oxygen monitoring is usually too labor intensive to be practical.

Progressive deterioration of oxygenation should be treated before frank hypoxemia develops. Verify ventilation and proper functioning of the endobronchial tube. Eliminate volatile anesthetic that may blunt hypoxic pulmonary vasoconstriction. Eliminate vasodilators that may blunt hypoxic pulmonary vasoconstriction. Apply oxygen with continuous positive airway pressure (CPAP) at 5 cm H_2O to the nondependent lung. Further adjustment of CPAP may enhance oxygenation. The nondependent lung may be reinflated with oxygen if necessary to achieve adequate oxygenation. If adequate oxygenation cannot be achieved, cardiopulmonary bypass should be initiated.

After surgical dissection, the pulmonary artery of the operative lung should be test clamped. Clamping of the pulmonary artery may improve ventilation-perfusion mismatch and oxygenation. However, severe pulmonary hypertension and right heart failure may develop. Vasodilators should be used to treat pulmonary hypertension and reduce right ventricular afterload. Inotropic support for the right ventricle may be necessary. The right atrial pressure should be monitored for evidence of tricuspid regurgitation associated with right ventricular dilation. Temporary unclamping of the pulmonary artery may be necessary to allow further pharmacologic therapy. If right heart failure cannot be controlled pharmacologically, cardiopulmonary bypass should be initiated.

Ventilation of the Transplanted Lung

After the lung has been transplanted, the pulmonary artery should not be unclamped until ventilation is possible. Perfusion without oxygenation of the transplanted lung would produce profound shunting and hypoxemia. The tidal volume should be adjusted to eliminate atelectasis and to achieve a peak inflation pressure of 20–25 cm H_2O with the chest open. The F_iO_2 of 1.0 is rapidly reduced in response to pulse oximetry and blood gas data. F_iO_2 is limited in the hope of curtailing free radical injury. PEEP may be used to enhance oxygenation. Hypoxemia is unacceptable.

Pulmonary edema may present a problem given the lack of lymphatic drainage. Diuresis and restriction of IV fluid may help. Mannitol and furosemide can be used to induce diuresis.

Typical total anesthetic doses for the entire intraoperative course:

1. Fentanyl 50–75 ug/kg or sufentanil 10–15 ug/kg
2. Midazolam 0.2 mg/kg
3. Vecuronium 0.3 mg/kg or pancuronium 0.2 mg/kg
4. Scopolamine 0.07 mg/kg

Postoperative Consideration

At the conclusion of operation, both lumens of the endobronchial tube should be aspirated and the tube should be replaced with a single lumen 8.0 mm (ID) endotracheal tube. Postoperative analgesia may be provided by infusion of narcotics through an epidural catheter. If cardiopulmonary bypass is used, the insertion of the epidural catheter should be delayed until normal coagulation function is documented in the intensive care unit.

Single-Lung Transplantation Operative Technique

Routine Single-Lung Transplant

The patient is then placed in a full lateral decubitus position. The chest, abdomen, and ipsilateral groin are prepped and draped in the operative field. A full posterolateral thoracotomy incision is made; a rib may be excised to improve exposure.

Single-lung ventilation is used if tolerated by the patient. Care is taken throughout the dissection to protect the phrenic nerve, and the vagus nerve with its recurrent branch. The inferior pulmonary ligament is divided. Both pulmonary veins are dissected and encircled outside the pericardium. The pericardium is opened immediately anterior to the veins and the pulmonary artery is encircled at its origin (dividing the ductus arteriosus on the left, if necessary). The main bronchus is encircled just proximal to its upper lobe division, taking care to preserve the proximal peribronchial lymph nodes and vessels.

The pulmonary artery is test-clamped to assess the hemodynamic response and oxygen saturation. Close communication with the anesthesiologist is critical at this stage. Normothermic cardiopulmonary bypass is readied if the patient is unstable with pulmonary artery clamping. The left femoral artery and vein can be cannulated for left lung transplant. Either the femoral vessels, or aorta and right atrium, can be used to establish cardiopulmonary bypass for right lung transplant.

Division of the hilar structures is done when the donor lung is available. All clamps are placed so they are out of the way of the surgeon, and so that they do not interfere with placement of the lung during implantation. The pulmonary artery branch to the upper lobe is divided first. The pulmonary artery is divided immediately distal to this branch. This allows increased pulmonary artery length, decreased size discrepancy with the donor lung, and the tie on the upper lobe branch aids in maintaining orientation. The veins are ligated and divided outside the pericardium, leaving stumps as long as possible. The main stem bronchus is divided just proximal to the upper lobe orifice (Figure 18).

The donor lung is prepared by dividing the bronchus two rings proximal to the upper lobe bronchus and preserving the peribronchial nodes and tissue. The pulmonary artery is mobilized from surrounding connective tissue at its origin. The atrial cuff is prepared, leaving at least 1 cm of atrium around the veins. A generous cuff of donor pericardium is brought with the donor specimen.

The donor lung is placed posteriorly in the chest. It is important to minimize handling of the lung. The table is rotated towards the operating

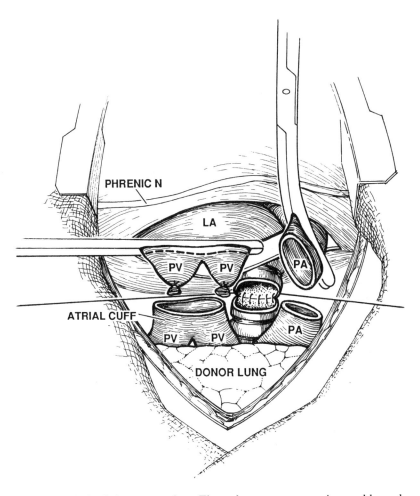

Figure 18. Left single lung transplant. The pulmonary artery, veins, and bronchus have been divided. The bronchial anastomosis is performed first with running 4–0 polypropolene.

surgeon to gain a better view of the hilum anteriorly. The recipient bronchus is trimmed two rings proximal to the upper lobe origin. There should be active bleeding from the cut edge that is controlled with cautery. The cartilage membranous junctions are identified to orient the donor and recipient bronchus. Running 4–0 polypropylene is used for the anastomosis (Figure 18).

A large curved vascular clamp is placed on the atrium with traction applied on both veins to maximize the size of the atrial cuff. Intrapericardial dissection of the pulmonary veins may be necessary. The atrial cuff is prepared by opening each vein and dividing the cleft between the vein stumps. The back and front walls of the atrial anastomosis are sewn from in front using running 5–0 polypropylene. The recipient pulmonary artery is clamped and trimmed to size. It is oriented by the tie on the first upper lobe branch. With pulmonary hypertension there may be a large size discrepancy, even beyond the upper lobe branch. This has to be compensated for while performing the anastomosis with running 5–0 polypropylene. The left atrial clamp is removed to allow back-bleeding into the pulmonary circulation and deairing is performed through the left atrial suture line. The lung is ventilated immediately to avoid hypoxia from shunting. Cardiopulmonary bypass, if used, is rapidly weaned, heparin reversed with protamine, and the patient decannulated.

The bronchial anastomosis, which usually retracts into the mediastinum, is surrounded by well vascularized tissue, and we do not use omental or other tissue wrapping. Meticulous hemostasis of the hilum is assured, and two chest tubes are used to drain the pleural space. The chest is closed in the routine fashion. An 8.0-mm endotracheal tube replaces the double lumen tube and fiber-optic bronchoscopy is performed to confirm a satisfactory airway anastomosis.

Single-Lung Transplant with Congenital Heart Defect Repair

For selected patients with congenital heart defects and Eisenmenger's syndrome, single-lung transplant can be combined with cardiac repair, instead of heart-lung transplant. This concept has been applied to patients with atrial septal defect (ASD), and patent ductus arteriosus (PDA), and could be applied to patients with a ventricular septal defect (VSD).

ASD closure and single-lung transplant is performed via right posterolateral thoracotomy. The patient is cannulated for cardiopulmonary bypass via either the ascending aorta or, if exposure is difficult, the right femoral artery. The SVC and IVC are cannulated. ASD closure is performed in the usual fashion with normothermic bypass. The heart can be fibrillated for a simple ASD closure, or the aorta clamped and cardioplegia given for more complicated defects. After ASD repair, the right lung is transplanted with the heart normothermic and beating.

A left thoracotomy approach can be used for the patient with a PDA. Partial bypass is established using the left femoral vessels. The PDA is divided in the usual fashion and left lung transplant performed. Alternatively, as reported from Toronto, the procedure can be performed via a median sternotomy, utilizing cardiopulmonary bypass. The PDA is closed after opening the PA anteriorly, and right lung transplant performed. Either median sternotomy with right lung transplant, or right thoracotomy with right lung transplant, could be used for VSD closure.

Indications for Cardiopulmonary
Bypass with Single-Lung Transplant

All operations for Eisenmenger's syndrome require CPB for single-lung transplant because of the cardiac repair and pulmonary hypertension. For patients with other causes of elevated PA pressure (e.g., PPH, pulmonary fibrosis with pulmonary hypertension) partial CPB should be used to decrease the PA pressure as much as possible. Clamping the dilated, thin-walled recipient PA for the anastomosis is much safer when it is decompressed. Finally, occasional patients with pulmonary fibrosis may be so hypoxemic that they require CPB for oxygenation. The capability for quickly instituting CPB should be present for all lung transplants, and it should be used if there is any concern regarding safe levels of oxygenation or pulmonary artery pressures.

Double-Lung Implantation

Patients with septic lung disease are considered candidates for double-lung transplant operation although, at Stanford, we have preferentially performed domino heart-lung transplant procedures until recently. The "classic" en block double-lung transplant operation was plagued by a high perioperative mortality, and problems with the tracheal anastomosis. We include this section on double-lung transplant for completeness; however, we currently prefer bilateral sequential single-lung transplantation.

"Classic" (en-bloc) Double-Lung Transplant

The operation (presented here for completeness, not used at Stanford) is performed through a median sternotomy incision with extension into the epigastrium for mobilization of the omentum. Cardiopulmonary bypass is always used. The pulmonary veins are stapled separately within the pericardium. The right and left pulmonary arteries are stapled, the left outside the pericardium to preserve the recurrent laryngeal nerve. The lungs are removed after the bronchi are stapled and divided, and the vessels are divided. The phrenic nerves are preserved on pedicles of pericardium as described for heart-lung transplant.

The heart is elevated and pericardial attachments to the posterior left atrium divided. The bronchial stumps are retracted caudally and, between the SVC and aorta, the distal trachea is mobilized and divided. The omentum is brought up through a small hole in the diaphragm, behind the heart, and placed next to the divided trachea.

The donor lungs are placed in the chest and the tracheal anastomosis is performed, then wrapped with omentum. Cardioplegia is given to arrest the heart and a portion of the recipients posterior left atrial wall excised.

The left atrial anastomosis is performed with running 3–0 polypropolene. Finally, the main pulmonary artery anastomosis is performed. The patient is weaned from CPB and decannulated in the usual fashion.

Bilateral Sequential Lung Transplant

This operation is performed through a bilateral transverse thoracosternotomy. Exposure of the pleural spaces is excellent and lysis of adhesions is therefore easier. First, the left lung is transplanted while ventilation is maintained to the right lung by way of a double lumen endotracheal tube. Partial cardiopulmonary bypass may be necessary. Ventilation and perfusion are then resumed to the transplanted left lung, and cardiopulmonary bypass can be weaned. The right lung transplant is then performed, frequently off bypass. After ventilation and perfusion are established to both lungs, cardiopulmonary bypass (if used and not weaned following the first lung transplant), is weaned. Postoperatively, an epidural catheter is very helpful for pain management.

Early Postoperative Care Following Heart-Lung and Lung Transplant

Routine Care

Postoperative monitoring and nursing routines are similar to post-heart transplant routines (see Chapter 3). However, heart-lung and lung transplant patients are kept in single rooms and strict reverse isolation procedures used (masks, gowns, and gloves/handwashing required of all personnel entering the patient's room). Low dose inotropic drug support is usually used for heart-lung transplants and patients with right ventricular dysfunction who undergo single-lung transplant. Isoproterenol or atrial pacing are used for heart-lung transplant patients to keep the heart rate 90–110. Hemodynamic management is typically even smoother than it is for heart transplant patients who had a low PVR preoperatively.

Immunosuppression

In brief, triple-drug immunosuppresion and induction therapy is used as for heart transplant recipients, but steroids are withheld from postoperative day 2 to 14 to facilitate bronchial healing.

Cyclosporine is begun 12–24 hours posttransplant when hemodynamics have stabilized and excellent urine output is established. If the patient has been extubated, oral cyclosporine is started at low dose (1–2 mg/kg orally BID) and the dose is adjusted according to daily cyclosporine level determination (target 150–200 by postoperative day 7). If the patient is intubated or in patients with cystic fibrosis who have impaired GI absorption, intravenous cyclosporine is started (3 mg/kg per day as a continuous infusion), monitoring daily levels, and this is switched to oral administration after extubation.

Azathioprine is given at 2 mg/kg per day (IV or PO). Early post-transplant there is frequently a leukocytosis (largely in response to perioperative steroids). This abates in a few days and if the leukocyte count declines below 5,000, the azathioprine dose is reduced.

Methylprednisolone is given IV (125 mg every 8 hours) for 24 hours (3 doses) posttransplant, and then steroids are withheld for 2 weeks. At that time, oral prednisone is started and 0.6 mg/kg in two divided doses and gradually weaned over a few weeks to 0.2 mg/kg per day. However, if there is evidence for rejection on bronchoscopy and biopsy (routinely obtained at weekly intervals early posttransplant) or on clinical grounds, IV steroid bolus "pulse" therapy (methylprednisolone, 1 gm IV daily for 3 days) and an oral taper is used, as in heart transplantation.

Induction therapy with OKT3 was routinely used at Stanford between 1987 and 1994. Briefly, 5-mg OKT3 is given IV for 2 weeks. T-cell subset monitoring and the details of the protocol are as described in the section on heart transplantation. Recently a short postoperative course of RATG has been given to all lung transplant recipients (2.5 mg/kg IV QD on postoperative days 1,2,3,5 and 7). This has been associated with fewer rejection episodes and improved survival at 3-years posttransplantation.

Respiratory Care

These patients should rapidly be weaned to an F_iO_2 of 0.4 or less to avoid oxygen toxicity to the transplanted lung. PEEP of 5 cm H_2O is routine, and occasionally has to be raised to decrease the percentage of inspired oxygen. The peak inspiratory pressure should be kept < 30 cm H_2O to avoid barotrauma (by adjusting tidal volume, PEEP, rate, etc.). Arterial blood gases are obtained every 1–2 hours during the initial 12 hours, then every 4–6 hours until extubated. Changes in pO_2, peak inspiratory pressure, or O_2 saturation need to be evaluated quickly. Suctioning the endotracheal tube should be performed every hour, and as needed, because bloody secretions may interfere with ventilation. Chest films are often taken every 12 hours for the first 2 days, then daily for the remainder of the hospitalization. The patient is actively diuresed as soon as possible after transplant. In addition, fluid infusions should be minimized and IV drips concentrated. Blood pressure is best supported by an infusion of dopamine at up to moderate doses, rather than by volume loading. Blood products should not be administered to correct abnormal coagulation parameters, unless bleeding is problematic. Perioperative fluid, blood products, the use of cardiopulmonary bypass, and divided lymphatic drainage of the transplanted lung all contribute to early postoperative pulmonary edema.

The patient is extubated when the hemodynamic condition is stable, there is no ongoing bleeding, the patient is awake and alert, oxygenation is acceptable ($pO_2 > 80$ mmHg on 0.4 F_iO_2), and ventilatory mechanics will allow for good gas exchange. Typically, this takes place 24–48 hours after transplant. Chest tubes are removed when drainage decreases and there is no air leak—usually 48 to 72 hours postoperatively.

Excellent respiratory care is extremely important early after extubation. Since the transplanted lung is denervated there is no cough reflex. This is specially important in heart-lung transplant patients in whom denervation extends proximal to the carina; these patients can develop copious secretions and not feel the need to cough. Incentive spirometry is helpful early postextubation, and throughout the hospitalization. Chest physiotherapy is applied every 4 hours to all patients for 48–72 hours postextubation. For patients who are too weak to cooperate, nasotracheal suctioning is occasionally necessary to help remove secretions. For patients with a single-lung transplant or a "clamshell" incision, an epidural catheter can be very helpful in allowing the patient to cough more effectively. This is placed in patients when the results of coagulation studies are normal. Finally, the patients are mobilized and ambulating as soon as possible.

Patients with primary or secondary pulmonary hypertension who undergo single-lung transplant have a large ventilation-perfusion mismatch. In many cases over 90% of the flow goes to the transplant but, in the early period, only 50% of the ventilation. These patients are at risk for rapid hypoxemia if secretions (or hemoptysis in one of our patients) impairs ventilation to the transplant. Therefore, after single-lung transplantation these patients should be positioned either supine, or with the transplanted lung up. If the transplanted lung is dependent they will have great difficulty clearing secretions and may become hypoxemic.

Postoperative Problems

Early Lung Graft Failure

Occasional patients will have poor immediate function of the grafted lung due to poor donor selection, inadequate preservation, or other perioperative problems (e.g., massive blood transfusions). This is manifested primarily by hypoxemia and the need for high levels of F_iO_2 and PEEP to maintain adequate oxygenation. The chest film typically shows diffuse pulmonary infiltrates and may resemble adult respiratory distress syndrome.

This clinical scenario has been referred to as the "reimplantation response" and is due, in part, to division of lymphatic drainage and edema of the transplanted lung. However, with the use of transbronchial lung biopsy in these patients, we have identified early changes (< 3 days from transplant) that appear to be due to graft ischemia with diffuse alveolar damage (see discussion of pathology in Chapter 11). Later onset of the "reimplantation response" (> 5 days) is more likely secondary to lung rejection (see Chapter 11).

The treatment of early lung graft failure is primarily supportive (diuresis, PEEP, increased F_iO_2). Rare patients in other programs have been briefly supported with extracorporeal membrane oxygenation. Early lung graft failure leads to prolonged intubation with a higher risk of nosocomial infection. In addition, lung graft rejection may be superimposed a few days later, thereby complicating the management even further. The outlook for these patients is guarded and underscores the need for careful donor evaluation and graft retrieval.

Cystic Fibrosis Patients

Cystic fibrosis patients typically have colonization of their sinuses with *Pseudomonas sp.* Despite preoperative antrostomies we have seen active clinical sinus infections within days after transplant. Because these upper airway infections can subsequently infect the transplanted lung they are treated aggressively. All cystic fibrosis patients are treated perioperatively with antipseudomonas antibiotics, as guided by sputum cultures, or empiric tobramycin. Irrigation of the sinuses with tobramycin is carried out at least monthly after operation. If there is active infection, drainage tubes are left in the sinuses for subsequent irrigation over several days. The participation of an otolaryngologist is critical for effective management of these potentially lethal infections.

The oral medication schedule of cystic fibrosis patients is more complicated because of poor gastrointestinal absorption. When oral intake resumes, pancreatic replacement enzymes are given as they were preoperatively. Typically, cyclosporine doses are higher than for most transplant patients, have to be given three times a day (instead of the usual BID dosing), and levels are harder to maintain in therapeutic range because of erratic absorption.

Gastric Stasis After Heart-Lung Transplant

Due to extensive dissection in the region of the vagus nerves many patients initially have poor gastric emptying after heart-lung transplant. It may be manifested by vomiting undigested food, a feeling of early satiety, and a large stomach seen on roentgenographic exam. Most patients improve with a short (2-week) course of metoclopramide. Rare patients have required prolonged treatment (see Chapter 12). Cyclosporine doses must be adjusted closely when metoclopramide is started as it rapidly increases serum levels.

Other Problems

Early cardiac dysfunction after heart-lung transplant is rare and is treated as outlined in Chapter 3. Other early posttransplant problems are as discussed in Chapter 4, and rejection and infection of the transplanted lung addressed in Chapter 11.

Selected References

1. Baldwin JC, Frist WH, Starkey TD, et al. Distant graft procurement for combined heart and lung transplantation using pulmonary artery flush and simple topical hypothermia for graft preservation. Ann Thorac Surg 1987;43:670–673.
2. Baumgartner WA, Trill TA, Camron DE, et al. Unique aspects of heart and lung transplantation exhibited in the "domino donor" operation. JAMA 1989;261: 3121–3125.
3. Benumof JL, Partridge BL, Salvatierra C, et al. Margin of safety in positioning modern double-lumen endotracheal tubes. Anesthesiology 1987;67:729–738.
4. Capan LM, Turndorf H, Chandrankant P, et al. Optimization of arterial oxygenation during one-lung anesthesia. Anesth Analg 1980;59:847–851.
5. Cavarocchi NC, Badellino M. Heart/lung transplantation. The domino procedure. Ann Thorac Surg 1989;48:130–133.
6. Cirella VN, Pantuck CB, Lee YJ, et al. Effects of cyclosporine on anesthetic action. Anesth Analg 1987;66:703–706.
7. Conacher ID, McNally B, Choudhry AK, et al. Anaesthesia for isolated lung transplantation. Br J Anaesth 1988;60:588–591.
8. Conacher ID. Isolated lung transplantation: A review of problems and guide to anaesthesia. Br J Anaesth 1989;61:468–474.
9. Cooper JD, Pearson FG, Patterson GA, et al. Technique of successful lung transplantation in humans. J Thorac Cardiovasc Surg 1987;93:173–181.
10. Eishi K, Takazawa A, Nagatsu M, et al. Pulmonary flow-resistance relationships in allografts after single lung transplantation in dogs. J Thorac Cardiovasc Surg 1989;97:24–29.
11. Egan TM, Detterbeck FC. Technique and results of double lung transplantation. Chest Surg Clin North Am 1993;3:89–111.
12. Fremes SE, Patterson GA, Williams WG, et al. Single lung transplantation and closure of patent ductus arteriosus for Eisenmenger's Syndrome. J Thorac Cardiovasc Surg 1990;100:1–5.

13. Griffith BP, Magee MJ. Single lung transplantation. Chest Surg Clin North Am 1993;3:75–88.
14. Hurford WE, Kolker AC, Strauss W. The use of ventilation/perfusion lung scans to predict oxygenation during one-lung anesthesia. Anesthesiology 1987;67: 841–844.
15. Jamieson SW, Stinson EB, Oyer PE, et al. Operative technique for heart-lung transplantation. J Thorac Cardiovasc Surg 1984;87:930–935.
16. Hardy JD, Webb WR, Dalton ML, et al. Lung homotransplantation in man. JAMA 1963;186:1065–1074.
17. McCarthy PM, Rosenkranz ER, White RD, et al. Single-lung transplant with ASD repair for Eisenmenger's syndrome. Ann Thorac Surg 1991;52:300–303.
18. Pasque MK, Cooper JD, Kaiser LR, et al. Improved technique for bilateral lung transplantation: Rational and initial clinical experience. Ann Thorac Surg 1990;49:785–791.
19. Patterson GA, Cooper JD, Goldman B, et al. Technique of successful clinical double lung transplantation. Ann Thorac Surg 1988;4:626–633.
20. Patterson GA, Tood TR, Cooper JD, et al. Airway complications after double lung transplantation. J Thorac Cardiovasc Surg 1990;99:14–21.
21. Reitz BA, Pennock JL, Shumway NE. Simplified operative method for heart and lung transplantation. J Surg Res 1981;31:1–5.
22. Reitz BA, Wallwork JL, Hunt SA, et al. Heart-lung transplantation: Successful therapy for patients with pulmonary vascular disease. N Engl J Med 1982;306: 557–564.
23. Sale JP, Patel D, Duncan B, et al. Anaesthesia for combined heart and lung transplantation. Anaesthesia 1987;42:249–258.
24. Scherer RW, Vigfusson G, Hultsch E, et al. Prostaglandin F2a improves oxygen tension and reduces venous admixture during one-lung ventilation in anesthetized paralyzed dogs. Anesthesiology 1985;62:23.
25. Schulte-Sasse U, Hess W, Tarnow J. Pulmonary vascular responses to nitrous oxide in patients with normal and high pulmonary vascular resistance. Anesthesiology 1982;57:9.
26. Shumway SJ, Burdive J, Bolman RM III. Combined harvest of heart and lungs: Technique and results. Transplant Proc 1991;23:1236–1238.
27. Siegel LC. Selection of anesthetic agent for thoracic surgery. In: Brodsky JB, ed. Problems in Anesthesia. Vol. 4. Philadelphia, JB Lippincott, 1990.
28. Siegel LC, Brodsky JB. Choice of anesthetic agents for intrathoracic surgery. In: Kaplan JA, ed. Thoracic Anesthesia. Second edition. New York, Churchill Livingstone, 1990.
29. The Toronto Lung Transplant Group. Unilateral lung transplantation for pulmonary fibrosis. N Engl J Med 1986;314:1140–1145.
30. Wyner J, Finch EL. Heart and heart-lung transplantation. In: Gelman S, ed. Anesthesia and Organ Transplantation. Philadelphia, WB Saunders, 1987, pp. 111–137.
31. Yacoub MH, Banner NR, Khaghani A, et al. Heart-lung transplantation for cystic fibrosis and subsequent domino heart transplantation. J Heart Transplant 1990;9:459–467.

Chapter 11

Rejection and Infection in the Transplanted Lung

Mordechai R. Kramer, M.D.,
Patrick M. McCarthy, M.D.,
Sara E. Marshall, M.B., B.S., Ph.D., MRCP,
Gerald J. Berry, M.D., Colleen J. Bergin, M.D.,
James Theodore, M.D., Bruce A. Reitz, M.D.

The morbidity of the lung transplant procedures exceeds that of heart transplants. Whereas episodes of cardiac rejection in the age of cyclosporine are most often asymptomatic and detected by routine cardiac biopsy, episodes of lung rejection are frequently symptomatic and sometimes rapidly progressive despite early treatment. Furthermore, in our experience, lung rejection occurs more commonly than heart rejection, and it occurs earlier after transplant. Cardiac rejection during the initial 2 weeks is very uncommon (see Chapter 6) and occurs in < 4% of patients on OKT3. However, lung rejection during the first 2 weeks occurs in > 50% of patients.

All transplant patients are at risk for developing respiratory infections. However, because of the denervated airways in lung transplant patients, and especially with denervation of the carina in heart-lung transplant patients, the cough reflex is diminished. The patients may develop secretions and not clear them effectively. This problem is compounded in patients with cystic fibrosis who frequently have colonization of the sinuses with Pseudomonas. Finally, the lung is the only solid organ that is transplanted that is constantly in contact with ambient air. This can lead to a wide range of fungal, viral, and bacterial infections in the immunosuppressed patient.

Immunosuppression

The same immunosuppressive regimen is used for heart-lung and lung transplant patients. Table 1 outlines the perioperative drug schedule

From: Smith JA, McCarthy PM, Sarris GE, Stinson EB, Reitz BA (eds.): The Stanford Manual of Cardiopulmonary Transplantation. Futura Publishing Co., Inc., Armonk, NY, 1996.

Table 1
Heart-Lung and Lung Transplant Immunosuppression

Immunosup	Pre-op/Intra-op	First 24 hrs	Days 1–3	Days 4–14	Maintenance
CyA	None	Start IV drip (3.0 mg/kg/day initially and when renal and hemodynamic fxn stable	IV drip to keep level 150–200	Change to p.o.	Level 150–200 1st 30 days 100–150 beyond
Azathioprine	4 mg/kg IV	2 mg/kg IV	2 mg/kg/day IV	2 mg/kg/day p.o. adjust for WBC <5,000	1–2 mg/kg/day p.o. adjust for WBC
Methylpredni-solone	500 mg IV intra-op	125 mg IV Q8 hours × 3	None	None (unless rejection)	For rejection episodes
Prednisone	None	None	None	None	0.6 mg/kg/day (divided bid); 0.2 mg/kg/day over 1 month
OKT3		Premedicate and give first dose IV drip (5mg)	Premed; IV drip; (5 mg)	5 mg IV push	If no antibodies may use for rejection episodes
RATG			2.5 mg/kg/day IV	2.5 mg/kg/day IV on days 5 and 7	May use for rejection episodes

and maintenance medications. Since 1986, patients have been maintained on triple immunosuppressive therapy including cyclosporine, azathioprine, and prednisone. Induction with OKT3 has been used since 1987. The major difference in this immunosuppression protocol as compared to the heart transplant protocol is that steroids are not routinely given during the first 14 days posttransplant. This is thought to allow better healing of the bronchial or tracheal anastomosis. The usual doses of methylprednisolone are given intraoperatively and for the first 24 hours. In practice, since lung rejection is common during the initial 2 weeks, bolus doses of methylprednisolone are given and we have not had any instances of airway dehiscence.

During the posterior mediastinal dissection in heart-lung transplantation, the vagus nerves may be injured and gastric stasis may be seen early postoperatively. Using intravenous (IV) cyclosporine (initial dose 3.0 mg/kg per day) provides a steady state infusion that could not be obtained with oral administration. Single-lung transplant recipients generally recover much faster and it is the surgeon's discretion whether to use IV or PO cyclosporine early posttransplant.

Lung Rejection

Clinical Presentation

Lung rejection may be insidious or may present quite dramatically. We have seen patients progress from appearing "well" on room air to requiring intubation and high levels of inspired oxygen within a 24-hour period. The clinician caring for these patients has to be acutely aware, therefore, of the signs and symptoms of lung rejection and quickly respond to any change in clinical status. The classic dilemma that frequently arises is the differentiation between lung rejection or an episode of lung infection. To make this important distinction we now rely on clinical signs and symptoms, chest film findings, and especially bronchoscopy with transbronchial biopsy for tissue, and washings for culture.

Several clinical features are typical of lung rejection. First, rejection frequently has its initial onset 7–14 days following transplant. Episodes of hypoxemia, pulmonary infiltrates, and dyspnea within the first 2 days after transplant are most often related to graft damage from the transplantation process (see Chapter 10). We have found lung rejection can occur early whether we use OKT3 for induction of immunosuppression, or RATG.

With the use of routine transbronchial lung biopsy, we have detected episodes of lung rejection in asymptomatic patients with clear chest films, but this is unusual. The most common clinical manifestation is a low-grade fever. This occurs in approximately 75% of rejection episodes. Patients usually also have dyspnea, and may develop tachypnea. Some patients will develop a feeling of malaise and have a mild nonproductive cough. The finding of a productive cough would be more suggestive of a lung infection than rejection. Hypoxemia, an increase in oxygen requirements, and decreased O_2 saturation (by pulse oximetry) also herald the onset of rejection (or infection).

Radiologic Manifestation

The postoperative chest radiograph may show multiple abnormalities that are commonly seen after thoracotomy. These include hemothorax, pleural reaction, fluid overload, pulmonary contusion, infiltrates, etc. There are, nonetheless, specific changes that occur with lung rejection. The most common chest radiograph abnormality during rejection episodes is the appearance of septal lines, subpleural edema, and peribronchial cuffing. Pleural effusions are also common during acute lung rejection and we have found the combination of new or increasing pleural effusion, together with septal lines to be highly suggestive of rejection. As rejection worsens, airspace disease can also be seen (Figure 1). The lower lobes tend to be involved more frequently than the upper lobes. In severe pulmonary rejection one may see bilateral interstitial and alveolar edema with bilateral pleural effusions (on some occasions up to several liters per day). Lack of pulmonary vascular engorgement and normal vascular pedicle width distinguish acute rejection from fluid overload or congestive cardiac failure.

The radiographic appearance of infection should be distinguished from lung rejection. Bacterial pneumonia is usually manifested by progressive segmental or lobar consolidation; cytomegalovirus (CMV) and *Pneumocystis carinii* pneumonia (PCP) usually present with bilateral perihilar interstitial or air space disease and uncommonly with pleural effusions. In many cases, however, lung rejection may be indistinguishable from lung infections, and tissue diagnosis is necessary in order to establish the final diagnosis.

In single-lung transplants, the transplanted lung is usually polygenic in contrast to the native lung and, therefore, venous engorgement is commonly seen. However, as in the heart-lung transplant patients, the appear-

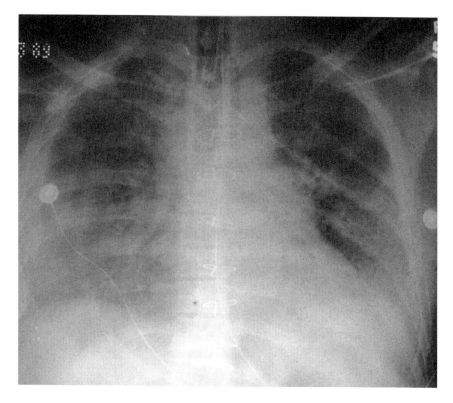

Figure 1. Chest film of a 43-year-old patient, 22 days following heart-lung transplantation for primary pulmonary hypertension. Bilateral airspace disease with septal lines and bilateral pulmonary effusions.

ance of septal lines or pleural effusion should raise the possibility of lung rejection (Figure 2).

Pulmonary Function Tests

Routine surveillance of patients posttransplantation includes close follow-up of the mechanical and physiological properties of the transplanted lung. The typical pattern after operation includes an initial decrease in lung volumes, which results in a moderate restrictive defect. This defect is thought to be related to chest wall abnormalities following surgery, donor-recipient size mismatch, and possibly abnormal lymphatic drainage. Over time this restrictive pattern improves progressively, and within 6 months

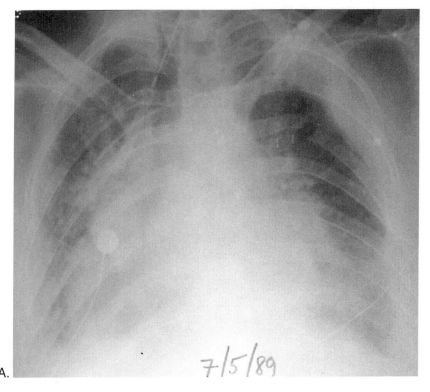

7/5/89

A.

Figure 2. Lung rejection in single-lung transplantation. (A) Chest film of a 35-year-old male 15 days post left lung transplant for idiopathic pulmonary fibrosis. Septal lines, pleural effusion seen on the left. Mediastinum is shifted to the right side. (B, see opposite page) Twelve days later following pulse with methylprednisolone and drainage of the effusion. Resolution of the rejection episode. Left lung is fully expanded with disappearance of the septal lines and most of the effusion.

lung volumes are close to predicted (recipient) normal values in most cases. Flow parameters in the immediate postoperative period are usually normal or slightly decreased in proportion to the low lung volumes. Arterial oxygen tensions improve dramatically following transplantation and gas exchange is near normal in uncomplicated cases.

Clinical and radiologic features, along with measures of gas exchange by continuous pulse oximetry and regular blood gas analysis, are used to monitor for acute lung rejection while the patient is in the intensive care unit (ICU). Once the patient is out of the ICU, spirometry and arterial blood gas measurement are obtained weekly. After the first month biweekly studies are performed for another 8 weeks, then monthly studies for the

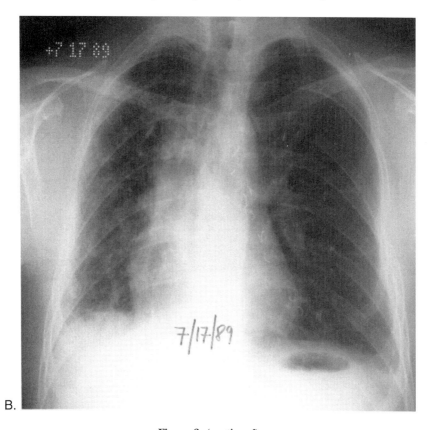

B.

Figure 2. (*continued*)

first year. Full pulmonary function studies including lung volumes, diffusion capacity (DLCO), and airway resistance are performed once every 3 months in the first year, and annually thereafter.

In our experience, the flow volume loop is a sensitive marker of pulmonary rejection. The forced expiratory flow rates between 25% and 75% (FEF_{25-75}) of the forced vital capacity (FVC) is particularly useful as it reflects alteration in flow dynamics of the small airways. These small airways are an initial target for the inflammatory response in lung rejection as demonstrated by morphologic studies in animal models and human recipients. A reduction of > 20% in FEF_{25-75} is highly suggestive of lung rejection (Figure 3). This is expressed by inward curving of the flow volume loop. Other parameters that may be reduced during rejection are forced expiratory volume in 1 second (FEV_1) and FVC.

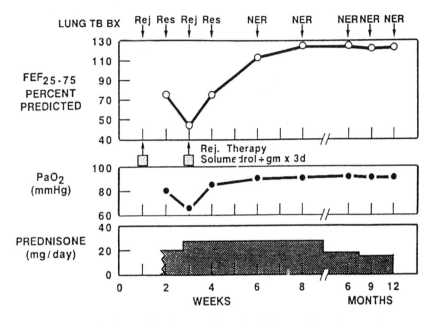

Figure 3. Lung rejection and pulmonary function. Changes in expiratory flow rates (FEF$_{25-75}$) and arterial oxygen tension during an episode of lung rejection (REJ), 3 weeks following heart-lung transplantation. Note improvement in hypoxemia and flow rates after steroid pulse. Repeated lung biopsy showed no evidence of rejection (NER). (Reproduced with permission from Starnes et al. J Thorac Cardiovasc Surg 1989;89:687).

Other centers may use FEV$_1$ as a guiding parameter but in our experience FEF$_{25-75}$ is more sensitive. Airway resistance may increase and diffusion capacity may decrease or remain normal during lung rejection. Although a decrease of FEF$_{25-75}$ is highly sensitive for lung rejection, changes in this parameter may also reflect an infectious process involving the airways as well. Therefore, following a significant drop in FEF$_{25-75}$ (> 20% decrease from baseline) immediate bronchoscopy is usually indicated and tissue and microbiological specimens are obtained. The obstructive changes of lung rejection rarely respond to bronchodilators but will usually respond to a steroid pulse (Figure 3).

In single-lung transplants, the flow volume loop may be less sensitive due to the fact that expiratory flows express combined function of both the transplanted and the native lung. However, similar changes have been observed in some of our cases with lung rejection.

Bronchoscopy and Transbronchial Biopsies

In conjunction with routine pulmonary function testing and chest radiographs, routine bronchoscopic examination with serial transbronchial biopsies improves the diagnostic capability for early detection of pulmonary rejection and lung infection. The protocol used at Stanford for bronchoscopic surveillance was formulated on the basis of previous experience, which demonstrated a high incidence of lung rejection in the first 3 months posttransplantation. Routine bronchoscopic examination with transbronchial biopsies are performed in weeks 1,2,3,4,8, and 12 posttransplantation. Later, bronchoscopies are performed at 6 and 12 months in the first year, followed by a routine annual bronchoscopy. Whenever rejection or infection is suspected on clinical grounds, bronchoscopy is immediately performed. Concomitant right ventricular endomyocardial biopsies are obtained in the heart-lung recipients during the first 3 months and annually thereafter.

Procedure: Bronchoscopy is usually performed under local anesthesia but general anesthesia may be indicated in some cases (e.g., pediatric patients). Antibiotic prophylaxis should be administered prior to the procedure. The procedure is performed under fluoroscopic guidance. The bronchoscope is passed via the nasal route except in patients with cystic fibrosis in whom the oral route is preferred in view of their prevalent sinus infections. After inspection, bilateral bronchoalveolar lavage is obtained. Lavage material is submitted for routine studies as outlined in Table 2.

Most tests are performed routinely; special tests (e.g., acid fast stain, tissue culture) are performed for specific clinical indication. Cell count analysis of the lavage fluid for the presence of lymphocytosis is used as a marker for rejection at some centers; this technique is not used at Stanford. Biopsies are performed with alligator forceps and at least 4–6 large pieces are obtained from one lung. The lower lobes are usually biopsied and several segments are sampled. If acute rejection or opportunistic infection is suspected, the biopsies are processed using a 90-minute rapid processing cycle ("Ultra"), and histologic sections are available within 3–4 hours. Routine biopsies are processed overnight.

Complications from bronchoscopy are rare and include pneumothorax and bleeding. In our experience with more than 300 bronchoscopies with biopsies in the last 3 years chest tubes were required in four cases for drainage of a pneumothorax; no episode of major bleeding or fatality has occurred.

In our experience, transbronchial biopsies have provided a positive diagnosis for either rejection or infection in about 52% of procedures. In some cases diagnosis was not clinically suspected and was first identified by the routine surveillance procedure. The introduction of routine bron-

---

Table 2

Specific Tests Performed on Bronchoscopic Specimens

A. Bronchoalveolar Lavage
1. Gram stain and bacterial culture
2. KOH stain and fungal culture
3. Viral culture
4. Shell vial monoclonal antibody stain for Cytomegalovirus
5. Acid fast stain and mycobacterial culture
6. Legionella direct fluorescent antibody stain and Legionella culture

B. Cytological Examination
1. Papanicolaou stain for CMV, herpes and malignant cells
2. Gomori-methenamine-silver stains (GMS) for Pneumocystis carinii
3. Cell counts and differential*

C. Protected Brush
1. Quantitative and anaerobic cultures*

D. Transbronchial Biopsy
1. Hematoxylin-eosin stain (H&E)
2. Elastic Van-Gieson stain (EVG)
3. GMS stain for Pneumocystis carinii and fungal elements
4. Acid fast stain*
5. Tissue culture*

---

*Optional, done in selected cases.

choscopy has significantly increased the detection of rejection episodes as well as infectious processes (Figure 4). Routine lung biopsies revealed lung rejection in 24% and pulmonary infections in 28% of 123 serial broncho-scopies, while routine cardiac biopsies were positive for rejection in only 16% of cases. It is important to remember that heart and lung rejection do not necessarily occur synchronously. In two-thirds of patients with acute lung rejection, there was no evidence of cardiac rejection. In contrast, in heart-lung recipients with heart rejection two thirds had concomitant lung rejection and in a third, lung biopsy was normal. Lung rejection is much more common than heart rejection in patients with heart-lung transplantation; the mechanism remains unclear.

Other centers have reported similar results with surveillance bron-choscopy with transbronchial biopsy and we consider it an important tool in longitudinal surveillance following transplantation.

The Pathological Changes of Lung Rejection

The morphologic manifestations of acute pulmonary rejection have been previously described in a wide variety of animal models. Studies in hu-

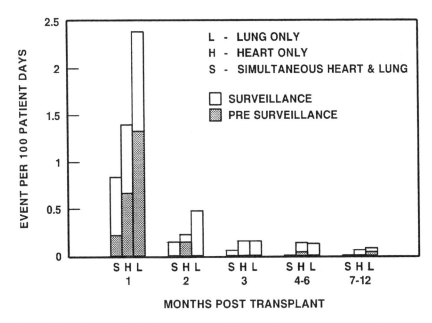

Figure 4. Incidence of rejection episodes following heart-lung transplantation. Incidence is highest during the first month and most commonly affects the lungs. Simultaneous heart and lung rejection occurs in less than a third of cases. The introduction of surveillance lung biopsies (open bars) increased significantly the detection of rejection episodes.

man unilateral lung and combined heart-lung transplants have suggested that the spectrum of morphologic changes mirrors those seen in the experimental models.

In the early phases of acute rejection (Figure 5) the peri venular tissue spaces are filled by transformed lymphocytes (immunoblasts), small lymphocytes, plasma cells, histiocytes, and occasionally eosinophils. A similar infiltrate is present in the peribronchial tissue and within the bronchiolar epithelium (mononuclear bronchiolitis). With increasing severity of rejection (Figure 6) denser mononuclear infiltrates are found around venules, arterioles, and bronchioles, within the endothelium of vessels (endovasculitis) and extending into the pulmonary interstitium. In severe rejection (Figure 7), massive bronchovascular and interstitial mononuclear infiltrates are seen with endovasculitis associated with vascular necrosis and thrombosis and pulmonary parenchymal damage. This may include alveolar edema, fibrin membranes, hemorrhage, and alveolar mononuclear exudates. The Lung Rejection Study Group recently presented a new formulation for the classification and grading of acute and chronic rejection (Table 3).

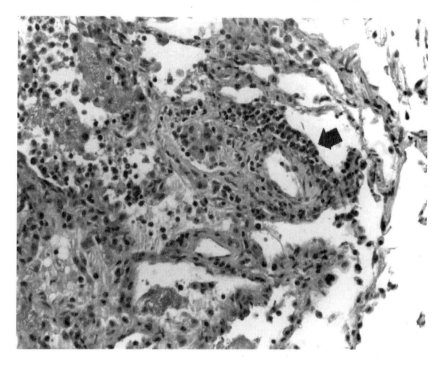

Figure 5. Mild acute rejection (Grade 2): sparse perivascular cuff of lymphocytes (arrow) intra-epithelial mononuclear bronchiolitis and minimal or absent endovasculitis (hematoxylin and eosin × 200).

A variety of morphologic entities may be seen within the setting of pulmonary transplantation that may mimic the changes of acute rejection both clinically and histopathologically. For this reason it is important that detailed clinical information accompany the biopsy specimen. Histologic entities that mimic the changes of acute rejection depend on the time interval from transplantation.

Graft Ischemia

Within the first 2–3 postoperative weeks changes related to graft ischemia may be observed. These range from patchy alveolar, interstitial, and intraepithelial accumulations of neutrophils, to diffuse alveolar damage (DAD) with fibrin membranes. Perivascular cuffing by neutrophils may occasionally be seen and the endothelium of vessels may display prominent reactive changes. Conspicuously absent are the mononuclear inflammatory infiltrates of acute rejection.

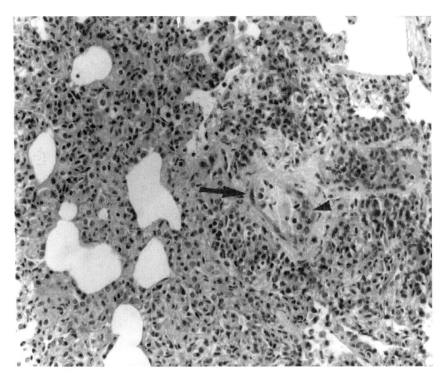

Figure 6. Moderate acute rejection (Grade 3): dense lymphocytic infiltrates around venule (arrow) with extension of mononuclear inflammatory cells into the pulmonary interstitium. Endovasculitis is seen (arrowhead) (hematoxylin and eosin × 200).

Artifact Distortion of Tissue

The transbronchial biopsy is susceptible to artifactual distortions from excessive manipulation that may lead to crush-related artifacts. These may be over-interpreted as evidence of increased cellularity and the inaccurate diagnosis of acute rejection.

"Bronchial Associated Lymphoid Tissue" (BALT)

Analogous to the gastrointestinal tract, the bronchial submucosa contains aggregates of lymphoid tissue that has become known as BALT. Their circumscribed arrangement, absence of the peri-vascular extension and inactive appearance of the constituent lymphoid cells allow discernment from acute rejection.

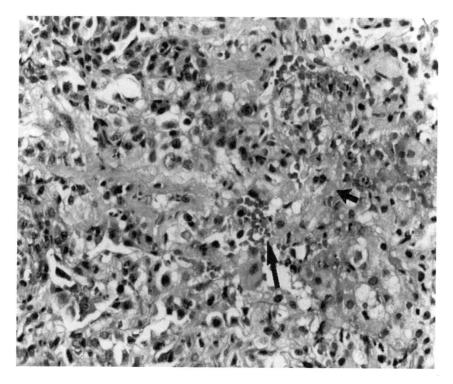

Figure 7. Severe acute rejection (Grade 4): alveolar parenchymal damage including fibrin membranes (small arrow), edema, mononuclear exudates and hemorrhage (large arrow) was seen in addition to the features of moderate acute rejection (hematoxylin and eosin × 400).

Biopsy Site Changes

Although less frequently observed than in endomyocardial biopsies, changes related to previous biopsy procedures may be encountered. They are composed of aggregates of fibrin, inflammatory cells, iron-laden macrophages, fibroblasts, and variable amounts of collagenous fibrous tissue. The absence of activated lymphoid cells and lack of bronchiovascular distribution are helpful diagnostic features.

Interstitial Mononuclear Pneumonitis

Interstitial pneumonitis may represent a nonspecific response to pulmonary injury and is occasionally encountered in transbronchial biopsy

---

Table 3
Working Formulation for Classification and Grading
of Pulmonary Rejection

A. Acute Rejection
   Grade 0 No evidence of rejection.
   Grade 1 Minimal rejection: Infrequent perivascular infiltrates not easily de-
           tected at low magnification
           a. with evidence of bronchiolar inflammation
           b. without evidence of bronchiolar inflammation
           c. with large airway inflammation
           d. no bronchioles present to evaluate
   Grade 2 Mild acute rejection: Frequent perivascular infiltrates that are easily
           observed at low magnification. Endovasculitis may be seen (Figure 5).
           a–d.
   Grade 3 Moderate acute rejection: Dense perivascular infiltrates with exten-
           sion into the alveolar septae. Endovasculitis is readily observed (Fig-
           ure 6).
           a–d.
   Grade 4 Severe acute rejection: Diffuse perivascular, interstitial and alveolar
           infiltrates composed of mononcuclear cells associated parenchymal
           damage. This includes necrotic cells, hyaline membranes, hemor-
           rhage and occasionally infarction or necrotizing vasculitis (Figure 7).
           a–d.
B. Active Airway Damage Without Scarring
   1. Lymphocytic bronchitis
   2. Lymphocytic bronchiolitis
C. Chronic Airway Rejection
   1. Bronchiolitis obliterans: Subtotal
      a. active
      b. inactive
   2. Bronchiolitis obliterans: Total
      a or b
D. Chronic Vascular Rejection
E. Vasculitis

(Reproduced with permission from Yousem SA, Berry GJ, Brunt E, et al. A working formulation
for the standardization of nomenclature in the diagnosis of heart and lung rejection: Lung rejection study group. J Heart Transplant 1990;9:593–601.

specimens. When associated with extensive airspace organization the histologic pattern resembles bronchiolitis obliterans with organizing pneumonia (BOOP-like). BOOP-like injury is likewise a nonspecific response and may be seen in a variety of settings, including ischemic changes, infections, and as a sequel of lung rejection.

Pulmonary Infections

Viral pneumonias may closely mimic lung rejection with interstitial and perivascular infiltrates of mononuclear inflammatory cells. The finding of cytomegalic or other viral inclusion bodies is an important diagnostic finding. As in the case of other solid organ allografts rejection and infection may coexist. In this situation we recommend a cautious approach with primary therapy for infectious process and early follow-up biopsies to evaluate for the presence of acute rejection.

Therapy for Lung Rejection

The initial therapy of lung rejection is bolus doses of intravenous methylprednisolone (Table 4). Steroids are given even though this may be during the initial 2-week period when we are trying to withhold steroids. We have not had any cases of bronchial or tracheal dehiscence and so feel comfortable giving steroids for rejection during this time. In an adult, for a severe episode of rejection, 1 gm of methylprednisolone is given every day for 3 days. If this is a very mild episode of rejection, asymptomatic, and detected solely by transbronchial lung biopsy, then only 500 mg a day may be given for 3 days. If rejection develops while the patient is an outpatient and has only mild symptoms and PFT changes, then we increase the oral dose of

---

Table 4
Escalating Treatment Options for Lung Rejection

---

1. Methylprednisolone 500–1000 mg IV Qd × 3, and oral prednisone taper.
2. Rabbit antithymocyte globulin Qd × 3–5 (3 mg/kg/day).
3. Repeat OKT3 (if antibodies negative) (5 mg/day).
4. Total lymphoid irradiation (2 ×/wk × 4 wks if WBC>3000); total of 800–1000 cGy.
5. Only as a *last* resort retransplant; or, if single-lung, transplant the contralateral lung.

---

prednisone to 50 mg PO, BID for 3 days with rapid tapering thereafter. Steroid boluses are used for the first and second episodes of rejection. Clearing of pulmonary infiltrates is sometimes dramatic within 24 hours, but more commonly resolution is slower. Within 24 hours, however, there should be improvement in the appearance of the chest film and the clinical condition of the patient. Approximately 80% of rejection episodes will respond to treatment in this manner.

For third episodes of rejection, or episodes that do not completely resolve, we give a 3- to 5-day course of RATG (see Chapter 6). Occasionally patients will develop refractory rejection and require further treatment. In such circumstances we have used a repeat 14-day course of OKT3 if antibodies to OKT3 are absent or the serum titer < 1:100. If OKT3 cannot be used, then we have used total lymphoid radiation (TLI) as outlined in Chapter 6.

Retransplantation is considered only as a last resort for severe refractory rejection. One pediatric heart-lung recipient underwent retransplantation for severe adenovirus pneumonia with refractory rejection. The patient died 1 month after retransplantation. We have not otherwise used retransplantation for acute rejection, but will consider this as an option. If this were being performed after single-lung transplant, then the option to transplant the contralateral lung would be considered.

Combined Heart and Lung Rejection

The treatment regimen outlined above is the same for either synchronous or asynchronous heart and lung rejection. If there is synchronous rejection of the heart and lungs and both are severe, we still follow the same treatment plan outlined above, but monitor the patient closely in the ICU.

Pulmonary Infections in the Transplanted Lung

General Aspects

Recipients of heart-lung or lung transplants are extremely susceptible to infectious complications and, in particular, pulmonary infections. Multiple factors may contribute to this susceptibility. First, the denervated lung has been shown to lack a cough reflex, a phenomenon that can often be observed during bronchoscopy when the bronchoscope is positioned below the tracheal or the bronchial anastomosis. Second, muco-ciliary clearance is abnormal in the denervated lung, as has been observed in radionuclide studies, and clearing of secretions and inhaled irritants is markedly impaired. Third, abnormal lymphatic drainage may also contribute to altered local clearing of secretions. Fourth, several investigators have shown that the transplanted lung has reactive airway hyper-responsiveness that may predispose to infection as well. Finally, the anastomosis site or any abnormal airway configuration (stenosis) may enhance local pathogenic colonization.

Rejection episodes result in increased susceptibility for infection because they usually require augmentation of immunosuppression. Moreover, during rejection the local inflammatory response with cellular sloughing and debris may serve as a potential medium for pathogenic colonization and subsequent invasion.

The donor lung may serve as a source of transmission of infectious agents, particularly in the case of those donors who have had prolonged mechanical ventilation. Grafts with previous quiescent granulomatous diseases such as tuberculosis, histoplasmosis, or coccidioidomycosis are susceptible to reactivation.

The recipient himself/herself may serve as a reservoir of infectious agents, especially when a single-lung transplant is performed. Moreover, for patients with cystic fibrosis, although the major source of infection (both lungs) has been replaced, residual sinus infections are very common, and local transmission of the infectious agent from the sinuses to the lungs is a major cause for morbidity in this population.

In the late postoperative course, the development of bronchiolitis obliterans or bronchiectasis may cause further airway injury and predisposes to chronic recurrent bacterial (commonly Gram-negative) infections.

In light of the myriad of predisposing factors, it is not surprising that respiratory infections comprise 85% of the total infectious complications in heart-lung and lung transplant recipients.

Importance of Lung Donor Cultures

Gram stain and KOH smear of the donor trachea are performed routinely to evaluate the donor for acceptability. Gram-positive bacteria are found in approximately 80% of patients and Gram-negative organisms in 35%. Earlier in our experience, yeast was present in 25% of the patients. The degree of colonization of the lungs depends on the length of time the donor has been intubated and possible aspiration near the time of death. Both at Stanford, and at Pittsburgh, there have been instances of early aortic suture line disruption, thought to be related to infection originating from the donor lungs. In the Pittsburgh experience this was closely associated with the findings of yeast on KOH prep. Because of this, most donors with significant amounts of yeast on the KOH prep are currently turned down as a heart-lung or lung donor. The presence of Gram-positive organisms on the gram stain has not led to clinically significant early problems and vancomycin is given perioperatively to the recipient. A donor who has been intubated for more than 48 hours, has many polymorphonuclear cells on gram stain of tracheal aspirates, and heavy colonization with Gram-negative rods would also be turned down for lung donation. However, small numbers of Gram-negative rods, with a shorter period of intubation, would not disqualify an otherwise acceptable donor, and we would use appropriate perioperative antibiotic coverage for the Gram-negative organisms.

Clinical Presentation of Lung Infections

Clinical presentation of pulmonary infections include fever, dyspnea, cough, sputum production, and occasionally chest pain. In heart-lung or lung transplant patients cough may be less prominent since the cough reflex is diminished below the airway anastomosis. Fever may be absent in patients on corticosteroids (unusual), and the white blood cell count may not be elevated because of treatment with azathioprine. Lung rejection may simulate an infectious process with fever, dyspnea, and new pulmonary infiltrate on the chest film. Physical examination is extremely important and tachypnea or a new auscultatory finding over the lung fields may suggest a possible infection. Spirometry may show decrease in expiratory flow rates and FEV_1, but may also be normal. Hypoxemia, or an increase in the A-a oxygen gradient may be the only abnormality in pulmonary infections such as PCP or CMV pneumonitis.

The chest film is helpful if a new infiltrate or nodular density is noted. Bacterial pneumonia is usually manifested radiologically as a unilateral airspace (alveolar) infiltrate, with or without consolidation. CMV pneumonitis or PCP commonly show bilateral interstitial infiltrates (Figure 8). Fungal infections can present in many forms, but a nodular presentation is more typical. Nocardia infection classically presents as a large nodular density.

A high index of suspicion is indicated when evaluating heart-lung or lung recipients and if a substantial possibility of lung infection exists, bronchoscopy with biopsies and cultures is done immediately.

Infection Surveillance

While the patient is intubated, daily tracheal aspirates are obtained for cultures and gram stains. Weekly viral cultures are obtained (urine, throat, and buffy coat), as well as weekly CMV serology for the first 2 months. As

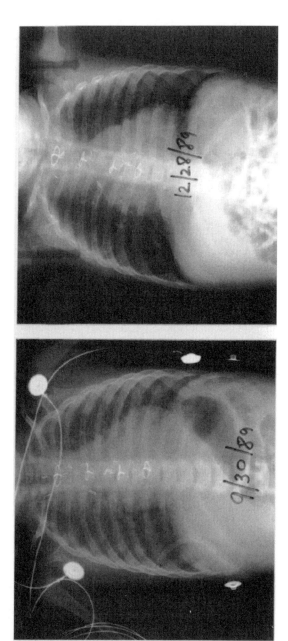

Figure 8. PCP. A 7-month-old child 3.5 months post heart-lung transplantation for Eisenmenger's complex presented with fever and cough. Chest film (left) shows bilateral increased interstitial markings. Bronchoalveolar lavage specimen yielded *pneumocystis carinii.* Chest film 3 months later (right) shows clearing of the infiltrates.

previously mentioned, routine pulmonary function tests and routine bronchoscopies with trans-bronchial biopsies may detect an infectious episode while the patient is asymptomatic. Not uncommonly, routine bronchoscopic examination may reveal a large amount of purulent material in the airways or positive cultures for pathogens in bronchoalveolar lavage or in lung biopsy in an asymptomatic patient.

Type of Infection

In a recent review of the Stanford heart-lung patient population, bacterial infections accounted for about half of all serious infections (Figure 9). Viral infections accounted for 30% of episodes; specifically, CMV was responsible for 16%. Fungal infections comprised 15% and protozoa infections (*P carinii*) constituted 5% of events. *Nocardia* occurred in 2% of episodes.

Overall, there were 188 episodes in 73 patients (average 2.57 episodes of serious infections per patient). Opportunistic infections account for about half of all infections.

Timing of Infections

The incidence of infection is extremely high during the first 3 months and decreases to a relatively stable rate after 1 year (Figure 10). Bacterial in-

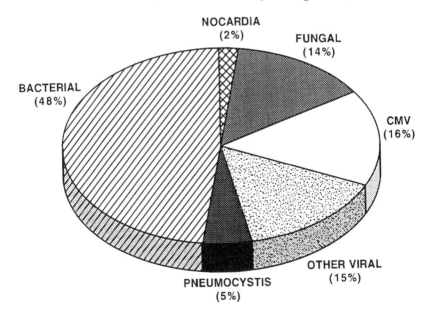

Figure 9. Infections in heart-lung transplant recipients: analysis of 188 serious episodes in 73 patients.

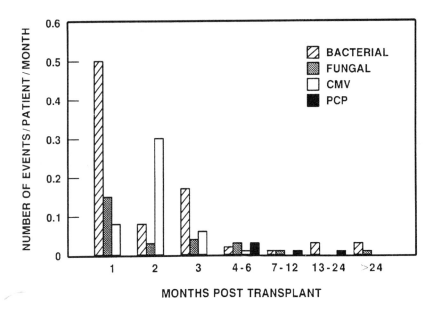

fections are the most common pathogens in both the early and late post-operative period. Viral infections are common between 30–120 days (e.g., CMV infections typically present in the second month posttransplant—average 42 days). Fungal infections usually occur in the first month post-transplant, but can present in the late postoperative course as well. Protozoa infections (PCP) occur most commonly 3–6 months postoperatively.

It should be remembered that whenever patients undergo augmentation of immunosuppression (e.g., for rejection episodes, bronchiolitis obliterans), increased vigilance for infectious complications is mandatory.

Specific Common Infections

Although pulmonary infections are more frequent in heart-lung transplants than in heart transplants, the clinical course and management of infections is similar. Several points should, however, be emphasized regarding heart-lung and lung transplant recipients.

Bacterial Infections

Nosocomial Infections.   As mentioned above, bacterial pathogens are the most common causes of infections in this population. Common nosocomial pulmonary pathogens include staphylococci and Gram-negative bacilli such as *Pseudomonas aeruginosa* and *Serratia marcescens*. *Staphylococcal bacteremia* that is usually related to intravenous line access, is also common during the immediate postoperative period. In the past, infection with *Legionella* was not uncommon in the first month posttransplant and routine cultures of bronchoalveolar lavage provide an accurate diagnosis. Direct fluorescent antibody stain (DFA) may provide rapid early detection.

Cystic Fibrosis Patients.   Heart-lung recipients with cystic fibrosis demonstrate a unique problem. Although the bulk of the bacterial load is removed during transplantation, foci of infection still remain in the sinuses and upper respiratory tract. In this population *P aeruginosa* is a common pathogen in both the early and late postoperative periods.

Preventive measures include surgical drainage of the sinuses (Cauldwell-Luc procedure) prior to transplantation with monthly tobramycin installation. Posttransplant irrigation is continued weekly. Despite these measures *P aeruginosa* is extremely difficult to eradicate and it is frequently cultured from sputum and bronchoalveolar lavage. Symptomatic bronchitis or sinusitis is treated with oral antibiotics, particularly ciprofloxacin, on an out-patient basis.

Late Bacterial Infections.   As will be discussed later (Chapter 12), one frustrating complication of heart-lung transplantation is the development of bronchiolitis obliterans. Chronic damage to the small airways increases the susceptibility to recurrent bacterial infections. Subsequently, with disease progression, bronchiectatic changes often occur in the lung bases with the resultant clinical picture typical of classic bronchiectasis, i.e., productive cough with large amounts of purulent sputum. The common pathogens include Gram-negative bacteria, mainly *P aeruginosa* and *Acinetobacter sp.* Eradication of these pathogens is extremely difficult and intravenous antibiotic therapy for 2–3 weeks may be required in the setting of severe infection.

Viral Infections

Cytomegalovirus Infections.   CMV infection is a common complication of heart-lung transplantation and may result from either reactivation of previous

Table 5

CMV Infection in Relation to Donor Recipient Status in Heart-Lung Recipients

	Donor −		Donor +	
	Infection	No Infection	Infection	No Infection
Recipient −	9%	81%	61%	39%
Recipient +	67%	33%	91%	9%

Infection defined as 3 fold increase in IgG titers, or new IgM, or tissue evidence of typical inclusion bodies.

latent infection in the recipient, or acquisition of the virus from the donor organs or blood products. Although matching for donor to recipient CMV status is routinely attempted, 60%–70% of seropositive recipients, and 60%–90% of patients receiving an organ from a CMV-positive donor, will show evidence of CMV infection. Infection is reflected by serologic studies (positive IgM or rise in IgG titer) or by overt clinical organ involvement, commonly pneumonitis. The Stanford experience is presented in Table 5.

Surveillance for CMV infection is performed routinely and includes weekly cultures of urine, throat, buffy coat, and bronchial lavage, as well as CMV serology (quantitative IgG and IgM). The clinical presentation of active pulmonary CMV infection includes fever, cough, dyspnea, leukopenia, and bilateral interstitial infiltrates on the chest radiograph.

Diagnosis can be obtained by serology, cultures, shell vial monoclonal technique, and tissue biopsy (gastric, colon, or transbronchial lung). The

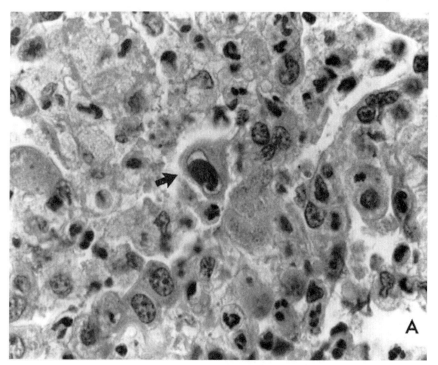

Figure 11. CMV pneumonia. (A) Classic CMV nuclear inclusion with large, homogeneous, eosinophilic to basophilic staining nucleus and clear zone ("halo") between the rim of the inclusion and nuclear membrane (arrow) (hematoxylin and eosin × 800). (B, see opposite page) Following DHPG therapy the intranuclear inclusions appear inhomogeneous, irregular in size and shape with absence of nuclear "halo" and fragmentation of the inclusions (arrows) (hematoxylin and eosin × 640).

most common histologic pattern is a diffuse interstitial pneumonitis (Figure 11A), although patterns ranging from minimal CMV pneumonitis with occasional inclusion bodies to diffuse alveolar damage have been observed. Immunoperioxidase and in situ hybridization techniques are useful in cases with equivocal histopathologic findings. Following the administration of gancyclovir (DHPG), there is alteration of the classic inclusion bodies with loss of the nuclear halo, fragmentation of the intranuclear inclusion, and irregularity of size and shape (Figure 11B).

Although CMV pneumonitis can be severe, in our experience in recent years, mortality is rare in the heart-lung or lung transplant patients. This may be accounted for by donor to recipient matching, early detection of infection by routine serologic, culture, or biopsy surveillance, and by prophylaxis with or early institution of gancyclovir (DHPG).

Prophylaxis with DHPG is used routinely for all seropositive recipients (5 mg/kg IV BID for 2 weeks, followed by 6 mg/kg IV daily for another 2 weeks), and also for a seronegative recipients receiving grafts from seropositive donors (5 mg/kg IV BID for 2 weeks, then 6 mg/kg IV daily for another 4 weeks). This prophylactic protocol is the same as the one used for

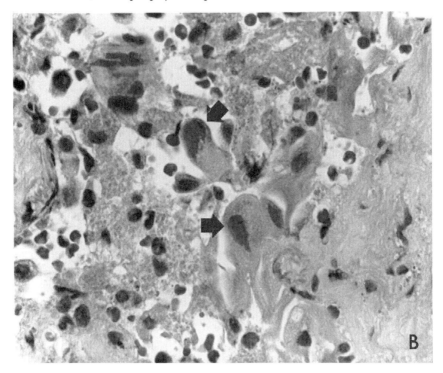

Figure 11. (*continued*)

heart transplants. Other centers utilize hyperimmune globulin and/or acy-clovir, which is given orally (but is much less active against CMV). CMV-negative blood products should be routinely used in CMV-negative recipients.

Bronchiolitis obliterans has been associated with previous CMV infections, although this relationship remains controversial. In some centers, long-term administration of anti-viral agents has been adopted. The patients may shed virus in urine or bronchoalveolar lavage fluid months and even years after infection while remaining asymptomatic.

Other Viral Agents.   Herpes simplex commonly occurs in the first month posttransplant and may cause oral ulcers or tracheitis. It usually responds to a short course of acyclovir therapy. Herpes Zoster usually occurs later and is self-limited in most cases.

Documented adenovirus infection has been observed in three patients; in one patient bronchiolitis obliterans subsequently developed.

Most patients undergoing transplantation have had Epstein-Barr virus (EBV) infection in the past, and reactivation may occur in the posttransplant period. Clinically, this has not been a significant problem except for the development of EBV associated lymphoproliferative disorders (Chapters 8 and 12).

Fungal Infections

Aspergillus Infection.   *Aspergillus sp.* has been cultured in about 25% of all heart-lung and lung transplant patients at Stanford. In five patients, disseminated invasive disease was found at autopsy. The delineation between infection and airway colonization is difficult and we tend to be aggressive in our approach to this situation. This attitude is based on our previous experience in which invasive/disseminated aspergillosis was found at autopsy in patients not suspected to have invasive disease.

Moreover, we have recently observed that aspergillus may cause severe tracheobronchitis with mucosal and cartilaginous invasion (Figure 12). Therapy usually includes amphotericin B, or more recently, itraconazole, a new oral antifungal agent that has been shown to be effective against aspergillus infections (see chapter 7).

Candida Infection.   *Candida albicans* commonly causes thrush in transplant patients. However, some patients may develop esophagitis, tracheobronchitis, and rarely pneumonia. Therapy should be preventive with topical nystatin. Severe candidal bronchitis or pneumonia is treated by administration of keto-conazole, fluconazole, or Amphotericin B.

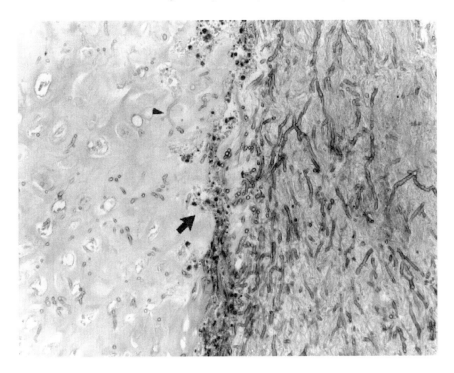

Figure 12. Aspergillus tracheobronchitis: dense infiltrate of aspergillus species hyphae with superficial erosion and necrosis of cartilage (arrow). Numerous branching septate hyphae are seen in the cartilage (arrowhead) (hematoxylin and eosin ×200).

Other Fungal Infections. Disseminated cryptococcosis has been found in one Stanford heart-lung recipient at autopsy; coccidioido-mycosis and histoplasmosis have been reported by other centers. Pretransplantation serological screening (see Chapter 9, Table 1), careful travel history, and aggressive therapy may reduce mortality from these uncommon but life-threatening infections.

Protozoan Infection

P carinii Pneumonia (PCP). The incidence of PCP usually peaks at 3–6 months posttransplant, but may occur later as well. The incidence of PCP in the absence of prophylaxis has been found to be as high as 88% in heart-lung transplant patients in one series. At Stanford only 15% of patients have developed PCP. The clinical presentation can vary from an asymptomatic state to severe respiratory failure. In contrast to the AIDS population, death from PCP in heart-lung transplant patients is rare, probably due to early detection by routine bronchoscopic surveillance studies (Figure 13). Since the introduction of prophylactic trimethoprim-sulfamethox-

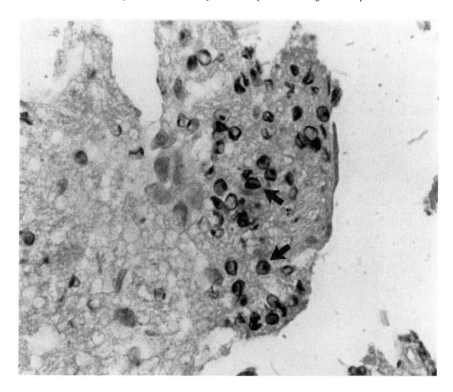

Figure 13. Pneumocystis pneumonia: alveolar exudates composed of foamy, loose proteinaceous material containing targetoid, helmut, and cup-shaped cysts (arrow). The microorganisms measure 6–8 microns in diameter. Cysts may also be seen embedded along alveolar walls. A variety of histologic patterns may be observed including classic pneumocystis pneumonia, interstitial pneumonia, granulomatous pneumonitis, diffuse alveolar damage, and interstitial pneumonitis with organizing pneumonia (BOOP) (Gomori's methenamine silver [GMS] × 800).

azole (TMP-SMX; 1 double-strength BID, 3 days a week), no patient has developed PCP while on prophylaxis therapy. Unfortunately, not all patients can tolerate the TMP-SMX prophylaxis due to gastrointestinal side effects or renal function impairment. Aerosolized pentamidine may be effective in such instances.

Other Protozoan Infections.   Reactivation of Toxoplasmosis has been seen in only one heart-lung transplant in Stanford, and is a less significant problem than in heart transplant recipients (see Chapter 8). *Giardia lamblia* was found in another transplant patient.

Other Infections

The incidence of nocardial infection in heart-lung transplants is 2%. It occurs late in the posttransplant course (up to several years) and may present with a lung mass. The introduction of TMP-SMX prophylaxis has probably reduced the incidence of disease due to this pathogen as well. Mycobacterial infections are uncommon in our population. In one patient, reactivation and subsequent dissemination of tuberculosis was observed. A dormant Gohn complex in the donor's lung may have provided the source of infection. In patients with previous tuberculosis the role of prophylactic antituberculous therapy is controversial, even when immunosuppression is instituted, since the source of infection (the lungs) is removed during transplantation. We do not advocate it.

Selected References

1. Brooks RG, Hofflin JM, Jamieson SW, et al. Infectious complications in heart lung transplant recipients. Am J Med 1985;79:412–422.
2. Burke CM, Theodore J, Baldwin JC, et al. Twenty eight cases of human heart-lung transplantation. Lancet 1986;517–519.
3. Burke CM, Glanville AR, Mackoviak JA, et al. The spectrum of cytomegalovirus infection following human heart-lung transplantation. J Heart Transplant 1986;5:267–272.
4. Cooper DAC, Novitzky D, Rose AG, et al. Acute pulmonary rejection precedes cardiac rejection following heart-lung transplantation in primate model. J Heart Transplant 1986;5:129–131.
5. Crumpacker C, Marlowe S, Zahng JL, et al. Treatment of CMV pneumonia. Rev Inf Dis 1988;10(Suppl):538–546.
6. Denning DW, Tucker RM, Hanson LH, et al. Treatment of invasive aspergillosis with itraconazole. Am J Med 1989;86:791–800.
7. Dowling RD, Baladi N, Zenati M, et al. Disruption of the aortic anastomosis after heart-lung transplantation. Ann Thorac Surg 1990;49:118–122.
8. Dummer JS, Montero CG, Griffith BP, et al. Infections in heart-lung transplant recipients. Transplantation 1986;41:725–729.
9. Gryzan S, Paradis IL, Zeevi A, et al. Unexpectedly high incidence of PCP infection after lung-heart transplantation. Am Rev Resp Dis 1988;137:1268–1274.
10. Harjula A, Baldwin JC, Starnes VA, et al. Proper donor selection for heart-lung transplantation. The Stanford experience. J Thorac Cardiovasc Surg 1987;94:874–880.
11. Higenbottam T, Stewart S, Wallwork J. Transbronchial biopsy to diagnose rejection and infection in heart lung transplant. Transplant Proc 1988;20:767–769.
12. Higenbottam T, Stewart S, Penketh A, et al. Transbronchial biopsy for the diagnosis of rejection in heart lung transplant patients. Transplantation 1988;46:532–539.

13. Keay S, Peterson E, Icenogle T, et al. Gancyclovir treatment of serious cytomegalovirus infection in heart and heart-lung recipients. Rev Inf Dis 1988;10(Suppl):563–572.
14. Millet B, Higenbottam T, Flower CDR, et al. The radiographic appearance of infection and acute lung rejection of the lung after heart-lung transplantation. Am Rev Resp Dis 1989;140:62–67.
15. Penketh ARL, Higenbottam T, Hutter J, et al. Clinical experience in the management of pulmonary opportunistic infection and rejection in recipients of heart-lung transplants. Thorax 1988;43:762–769.
16. Pollard RB. Cytomegalovirus infections in renal, heart, heart-lung and liver transplantation. Pediatr Inf Dis J 1988;7:97–112.
17. Reitz BA, Guadiani VA, Hunt SA, et al. Diagnosis and treatment of allograft rejection in heart-lung transplant recipients. J Thorac Cardiovasc Surg 1983;85: 354–361.
18. Starnes VA, Theodore J, Oyer PE, et al. Evaluation of heart lung transplant recipients with prospective serial transbronchial biopsies and pulmonary function studies. J Thorac Cardiovasc Surg 1989;98:683–690.
19. Starnes VA, Theodore J, Oyer PE, et al. Pulmonary infiltrates after heart-lung transplantation: Evaluation by serial transbronchial biopsies. J Thorac Cardiovasc Surg 1989;98:945–950.
20. Stewart S, Higenbottam T, Hutter JA, et al. Histopathology of transbronchial biopsies in heart-lung transplantation. Transplant Proc 1988;20:764–766.
21. Tazelaar HD, Baird AM, Mill M, et al. Bronchocentric mycosis occurring in transplant recipients. Chest 1989;96:92–95.
22. Theodore J, Jamieson SW, Burke CM, et al. Physiologic aspects of human heart-lung transplantation. Chest 1984;86:349–357.
23. Yousem SA. Am J Surg Pathol 1992;16:877–884.
24. Yousem SA, Berry GJ, Brunt E, et al. A working formulation for the standardization of nomenclature in the diagnosis of heart and lung rejection: Lung rejection study group. J Heart Transplant 1990;9:593–601.
25. Zeevi A, Fung JJ, Paradis IL, et al. Lymphocytes of bronchoalveolar lavage from heart-lung transplant recipients. Heart Transplant 1985;4:417–421.
26. Zenati M, Dowling RD, Armitage JM, et al. Organ procurement for pulmonary transplantation. Ann Thorac Surg 1989;48:882–886.

Chapter 12

Late Complications and Results in Heart-Lung and Lung Transplantation and Future Directions in Cardiopulmonary Transplantation

Mordechai R. Kramer, M.D.,
Julian A. Smith, M.B., M.S., FRACS,
Patrick M. McCarthy, M.D., Gerald J. Berry, M.D.,
Sara E. Marshall, M.B., B.S., Ph.D., MRCP,
James Theodore, M.D., Norman J. Lewiston, M.D.

The majority of operative complications, episodes of acute rejection, and most infections occur in the first 6 months following transplantation. The routine follow-up after this period is intended to detect infections, monitor effects (and side effects) of immunosuppression therapy, monitor for systemic complications or unrelated disease, and detect the development of bronchiolitis obliterans as early as possible.

Follow-up is performed monthly in the first year, and bimonthly thereafter, by the referring physician in close association with the transplant team. The monthly checkup should include physical examination, chest film, spirometry, arterial blood gases, and laboratory work (blood count, electrolytes, renal and hepatic panels, and cyclosporine levels). Annual studies are performed at the transplantation center and include: bronchoscopy with transbronchial biopsy, echocardiography, cardiac catheterization with right heart biopsy, and coronary angiogram (for heart-lung transplant patients), chest computed tomography (CT) scan, and full pulmonary function tests. Single and double lung transplant patients also have MUGA scans to assess right and left ventricular ejection fractions and sin-

From: Smith JA, McCarthy PM, Sarris GE, Stinson EB, Reitz BA (eds.): The Stanford Manual of Cardiopulmonary Transplantation. Futura Publishing Co., Inc., Armonk, NY, 1996.

263

Table 1

Late Complications After Heart-Lung and Lung Transplantation

A. Pulmonary Disorders
   1. Lung infections
   2. Bronchiolitis obliterans
   3. Bronchiectasis
   4. Airway complications
B. Accelerated Coronary Artery Disease
C. Complications Related to Immunosuppressive Drugs
   1. Hypertension
   2. Chronic renal failure
   3. Hyperuricemia/Gout
   4. Hypercholesterolemia
   5. Hypercortisolism
   6. Lymphoproliferative disorders (lymphoma)
   7. Anemia, leukopenia, thrombocytopenia
D. Skin Disorders
   1. Acne vulgaris
   2. Papillomata
   3. Subcutaneous masses
   4. Skin cancer
E. Gastric Dysmotility
F. Psychological Disorders
G. Neurological Disorders
   1. Pseudo-tumor cerebri
   2. CNS infections
H. Diabetes Mellitus
I. Liver Dysfunction
   1. Raised liver enzymes
   2. Hepatitis C

gle lung patients undergo ventilation/perfusion scanning. For this purpose the patient is admitted for 3–4 days and additional studies and consultation are performed as necessary. The major late complications are described in Table 1.

Late Complications

Many of the drug-induced complications are discussed in chapters dealing with heart transplant recipients (Chapters 6, 7, and 8). Here, we will try to review the major complications more specific to the patients with a heart-lung and lung transplant.

Obliterative Bronchiolitis

Definition

Obliterative bronchiolitis (OB) is a rapidly progressive inflammatory disorder of unknown etiology that attacks the small airways of the transplanted lung and causes severe, often irreversible, obstructive lung disease.

Etiology

Several hypotheses have been postulated for the pathogenesis of this syndrome. Chronic rejection is thought to be an important mechanism as lymphocytes accumulate in the submucosa of the inflamed airways. Enhanced expression of major histocompatibility antigens Class I and II has been found in endothelial as well as epithelial cells from lungs with OB. Furthermore, in some cases both physiologic and pathologic changes have responded to augmented immunosuppression implying that rejection is a possible mechanism. Human lymphocyte antigen (HLA) mismatch, particularly at more than one locus, has also been associated with a higher incidence of the syndrome while a match in the A locus seems to have a protective effect on the development of OB. A similar syndrome was found as part of graft versus host disease in bone marrow transplant, suggesting an immunologically mediated response targeted at the small airways.

Infections have also been implicated as a possible etiology for the inflammatory reaction attacking the small airways. A high incidence of preceding infections with cytomegalovirus (CMV) or *Pneumocystis carinii* has been reported in association with OB. In many instances deterioration of lung function was preceded by an upper respiratory tract infection. In some cases influenza virus, adenovirus, and respiratory syncytial virus infection were found in association with the development of the disease.

Lung denervation and the loss of the bronchial circulation may play a role in the damage to the small airways and resultant bronchiolitis. It is possible, as suggested by Burke et al., that a combination of factors leads to this destruction process. A viral infection may trigger the rejection process by amplification of the antigenic expression in the small airways. The lack of proper blood supply may prevent the normal healing response. Overall, at this point in time, there is no clear insight into the pathogenesis of this devastating complication.

Incidence and Timing Posttransplant

The incidence of OB varies from series to series but occurs in 10%–54% of heart-lung transplant recipients and to a lesser extent among single lung transplant recipients. Following the first 101 heart-lung transplants at Stanford, the incidence of OB was 28% at 1 year, 45% at 5 years, and 53% at 10 years posttransplant. Of 33 single or double-lung transplants, the incidence of OB was 17% at 3-years posttransplant. During the period 1981–1986 when the immunosuppressive regimen for heart-lung transplantation consisted only of cyclosporine and prednisone, the incidence of OB (63%) was twice that observed between 1986 and 1994 (33%) when triple therapy (cyclosporine, prednisone, azathioprine) was used. The disease may develop at any time posttransplantation, but is most commonly recognized towards the end of the first year (mean 10 months; Figure 1).

Clinical Manifestation

The deterioration of lung function associated with OB may be rapid, or the onset of the disease may be insidious. A mild upper respiratory syndrome may occur with fever and dry cough. Progressive dyspnea occurs

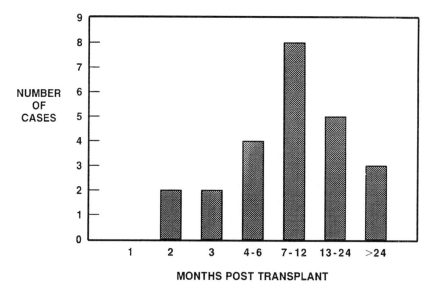

Figure 1. Timing of occurrence of OB following transplantation.

within several weeks. Physical examination may reveal fine inspiratory crepitations (squeaks) with occasional wheezing. With disease progression recurrent infections are frequent and bronchiectatic changes may develop. The chest film is frequently not helpful in the diagnosis of OB as it may remain clear even when the disease is far advanced. Radiographic changes may include peribronchial, and occasional interstitial infiltrates, mainly in lung bases. Bronchiectatic changes may sometimes be seen on CT scans, and bronchial dilatation on high resolution CT scans may be an indication of OB.

Pulmonary Function Testing

In OB, serial measurements of pulmonary function reveal progression of severe obstructive lung disease. Airflow is markedly decreased with reduction in FEV_1 and expiratory flow rates to extremely low values (Figure 2). The shape of the flow volume loop shows inward caving of the loop with rapid decrease in flow rate and forced expiratory volume developing over several months. In contrast to classic changes of chronic obstructive pulmonary disease (i.e., emphysema) in which there is air trapping and increased lung volumes, in OB the lung volumes (total lung capacity, func-

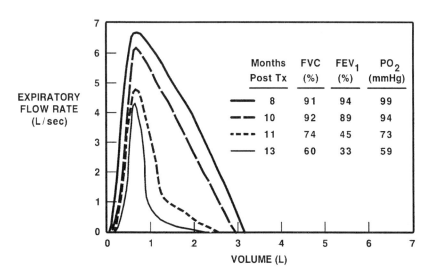

Months Post Tx	FVC (%)	FEV_1 (%)	PO_2 (mmHg)
—— 8	91	94	99
– – 10	92	89	94
···· 11	74	45	73
—— 13	60	33	59

Figure 2. Pulmonary function in OB: note the rapid deterioration over 2 months in shape of flow-volume loop, forced vital capacity (FVC), expiratory flow rates (FEV_1), and arterial oxygen tension (PO_2).

tional residual capacity, residual volume) are most often reduced, thus demonstrating a coexisting progressive restrictive pattern. Diffusion capacity of carbon monoxide is often moderately reduced and airway resistance markedly increased. Arterial blood gases shows progressive hypoxemia with hypocapnia and an increase in the alveolar-arterial oxygen tension gradient (A-a gradient). Response to bronchodilators is usually absent or minimal.

Pathological Changes

A morphologic spectrum of changes have been observed in OB that reflect the development and evolution of the necrotizing inflammatory process. In the early stages, a mononuclear infiltrate is observed in the mucosal and muscular layers of the airways. Following epithelial damage, there

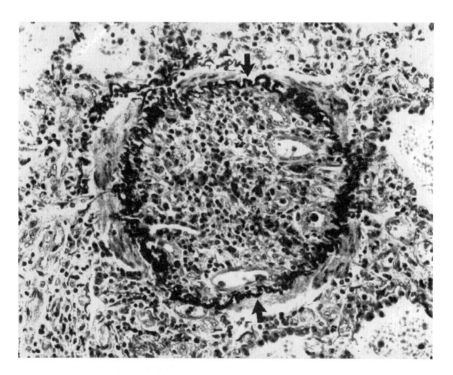

Figure 3. Obliterative bronchiolitis: intraluminal aggregates of necrotic and displaced bronchiolar epithelial lining cells admixed with dense inflammatory infiltrate composed of lymphocytes, plasma cells, and occasional histiocytes. The elastic lamina of the bronchiole remains intact in the early stages of bronchiolar inflammation and injury (arrow) (elastic-von-Gieson × 125).

is necrosis and sloughing of cells into the lumina of the respiratory and terminal bronchioles and alveolar ducts. Mucosal ulceration with a mononuclear or mixed inflammatory response is often seen. Organization occurs (Figure 3) with development of granulation tissue plugs (Masson bodies). Fibroblasts, macrophages, and other inflammatory cells are activated leading to the development of fibrous scarring in the submucosal layers. The diagnosis of OB may be difficult on routine hematoxylin and eosin sections and we find the use of an elastic stain (e.g., EUG) to be helpful in difficult cases. These may subsequently undergo incomplete or total resorption with partial or complete restoration of the lumen, or may progress to fibrotic occlusion (Figure 4) of the lumen. The Lung Rejection Study Group has recently proposed a new classification of OB that reflects the degree of inflammation and damage of the airways (Table 2). Augmentation of immunosuppressive therapy may arrest or reverse the early stages, but not

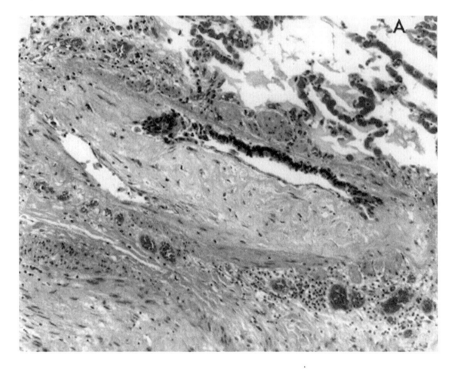

Figure 4. OB. (A) Late stages of OB with near complete occlusion of the bronchiolar lumen by fibrous scar tissue, partial epithelial sloughing and submucosal fibrosis (hematoxylin and eosin × 125). (B, see opposite page) The EVG stain highlights the degree of luminal narrowing, disruption of bronchiolar elastica (large arrow), and atrophy of the muscular layer small arrow) (elastic von Gieson × 125).

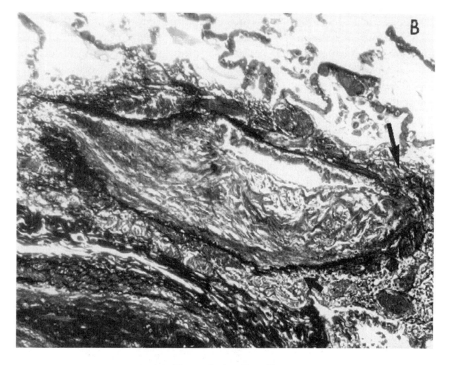

Figure 4. *(continued)*

the late changes. The transbronchial biopsy may be helpful in document-ing the presence of OB; however, the process is patchy in nature and tissue sampling error must be considered in patients with physiologic changes suggestive of OB.

Diagnosis

Early detection of the disease by pulmonary function testing is ex-tremely important because in some patients augmentation of immunosup-pressive therapy, early in the course, has been shown to improve lung func-tion and arrest the destructive process. Close monitoring of the flow-volume loop during the months posttransplantation is needed. In our experience, a significant reduction in flow rates, in particular FEF_{25-75}, may imply the development of OB. This parameter (FEF_{25-75}) is probably an early indicator of damage to the target of the inflammatory process (i.e., the small airways) and falls earlier than other flow parameters (FEV_1).

Table 2
Working Formulation for Classification and Grading
of Pulmonary Rejection

A. Acute Rejection
   Grade 0 No evidence of rejection.
   Grade 1 Minimal rejection: Infrequent perivascular infiltrates not easily detected at low magnification
      a. with evidence of bronchiolar inflammation
      b. without evidence of bronchiolar inflammation
      c. with large airway inflammation
      d. no bronchioles present to evaluate
   Grade 2 Mild acute rejection: Frequent perivascular infiltrates that are easily observed at low magnification. Endovasculitis may be seen.
      a–d.
   Grade 3 Moderate acute rejection: Dense perivascular infiltrates with extension into the alveolar septae. Endovasculitis is readily observed.
      a–d.
   Grade 4 Severe acute rejection: Diffuse perivascular, interstitial and alveolar infiltrates composed of mononcuclear cells associated parenchymal damage. This includes necrotic cells, hyaline membranes, hemorrhage and occasionally infarction or necrotizing vasculitis.
      a–d.
B. Active Airway Damage Without Scarring
   1. Lymphocytic bronchitis
   2. Lymphocytic bronchiolitis
C. Chronic Airway Rejection
   1. Bronchiolitis obliterans: Subtotal
     a. active
     b. inactive
   2. Bronchiolitis obliterans: Total
     a. or b.
D. Chronic Vascular Rejection
E. Vasculitis

(Reproduced with permission from Yousem SA, Berry GJ, Brunk EM; et al. A working formulation for the standardization of nomenclature in the diagnosis of heart and lung rejection: Lung rejection study group. J Heart Transplant 1990;9:593–601.

Bronchoscopy with transbronchial biopsies is usually performed at this point and infection or acute rejection ruled out. Since disease is focal in nature, transbronchial biopsy may not always be diagnostic and commonly diagnosis is made merely on physiologic grounds (Figure 5).

Prevention and Therapy

As the etiology of OB is unclear, prevention is difficult to achieve. Improved immunosuppression regimens with triple drug therapy (cyclosporine, azathioprine, prednisone) may reduce the incidence of OB. The correlation between previous airway damage by infectious processes (PCP, CMV, and other viruses) and OB suggests that an aggressive approach toward infections may decrease this complication. Once OB is clinically suspected a trial of increased immunosuppression is indicated and a pulse of prednisone to 1 mg/kg is given for 1 week and then tapered down over several weeks. Success in reversing the disease has been documented but experience is limited. In many instances disease may progress despite therapy.

Prognosis

Since 1986, patients on triple immunosuppressive therapy have been shown to have a lower incidence of OB with reduced mortality from the disease. Disease severity has also been reduced and long-term survivors are now followed 4–6 years after developing OB. Once the disease turns into its chronic form, patients tend to develop bronchiectatic changes with recurrent infections. Therapy then includes antibiotics, bronchodilators, and rigorous pulmonary toilet. In advanced cases oxygen supplementation may be required. End-stage patients may be candidates for retransplantation and single-lung transplantation is the procedure of choice, unless bronchiectasis and recurrent infections are common.

Proximal Bronchiectasis

Previous postmortem studies have shown the coexistence of OB with large airway inflammation and dilatation (Figure 6). Alternating changes of dilatation and narrowing of the bronchial tree are seen macroscopically and by bronchogram studies. Chronic inflammation, mucosal sloughing and luminal plugs of mucus, and atrophy of the muscle of the bronchi are

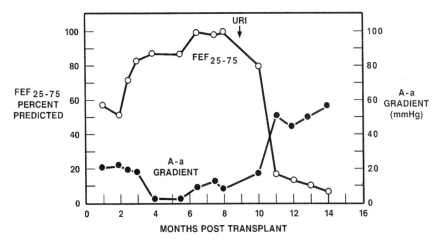

Figure 5. OB: the changes in forced expiratory flow rates between 25%–75% of the forced vital capacity (FEF$_{25-75}$) and alveolar-arterial (A-a) gradient. URI denotes upper respiratory tract infection, which preceded the occurrence of the disease.

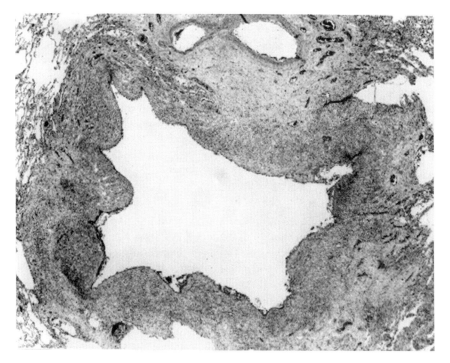

Figure 6. Proximal bronchiectasis: large airway inflammation and dilatation in a combined heart-lung recipient with coexistent OB (hematoxylin and eosin × 30).

the major histopathological features. Whether these changes represent the results of mechanical obstruction or a form of chronic rejection remain unknown. Clinically, patients present with recurrent infections and often heavy sputum production. Pulmonary function tests shows obstructive and restrictive changes and CT scan may be helpful in diagnosis. Only retransplantation of both lungs can be offered for therapy.

Other Late Complications

Bronchial Stenosis

Several centers have reported the development of bronchial anastomotic site stenosis posttransplant. This complication occurred as a result of ischemic changes from the interruption of bronchial blood supply during transplantation. Wrapping the anastomotic site with omentum reduced the rate of bronchial stenosis by providing an alternative blood supply. A very low incidence of bronchial stenosis has been observed when the recipient bronchus was "telescoped" inside that of the donor as a part of the anastomotic technique. Many groups, including ourselves, no longer wrap the anastomosis with omentum. In our single and bilateral sequential lung transplant population there have been only three cases of bronchial stenosis. The first was managed by dilatation with the rigid bronchoscope, the second by balloon dilatation, and the third by laser debulking of granulation tissue followed by the insertion of an expandable metal stent.

Ventilation-Perfusion Mismatches

Theoretically, transplantation of a healthy lung with normal mechanical properties juxtaposed to a diseased lung will cause inequality of distribution of ventilation and perfusion. In patients with pulmonary fibrosis the problem is minimal since the lower compliance of the native lung will shift ventilation to the new lung and the slightly higher pulmonary vascular resistance in the native lung will shift most of perfusion to the transplanted lung as well (Figure 7).

In contrast, theoretically, transplantation of a single lung in emphysema, with higher compliance of the native lung, may cause reduced ventilation to the transplanted lung. In practice, patients with emphysema who have re-

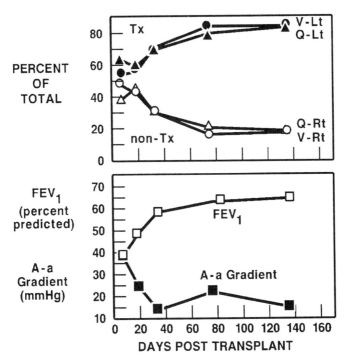

Figure 7. Ventilation (V) and perfusion (Q) distribution following uncomplicated single-lung transplantation (left lung) for idiopathic pulmonary fibrosis. Upper graph, the transplanted lung (Tx) (top) receives 80% of both V and Q, 140 days following transplantation. The native lung (non-Tx) get only 20% of the total. This results (lower graph) in excellent gas exchange with normal alveolar-arterial (A-a) gradient. Forced expiratory volume in 1 second (FEV_1) improved significantly following transplantation and reaches 70% of predicted value.

ceived a single lung transplant have shown hyperinflation of the old lung but have maintained good gas exchange with progressive V/Q matching.

In patients with pulmonary hypertension the perfusion shifts almost immediately to the low resistance, transplanted lung while ventilation initially remains evenly distributed. This V/Q mismatch may lead to mild to moderate hypoxemia and in the immediate postoperative period patients may have to be positioned to improve ventilation in the new lung. Over time, there is a gradual shift of ventilation to the transplanted side and better V/Q matching. This is probably due to bronchoconstrictor reflexes secondary to decreased local blood flow and hypocarbia in the native lung.

During rejection episodes, we have noticed that ventilation shifts to the native side with resulting arterial hypoxemia. When rejection worsens and vascular resistance rises, perfusion may also shift to the native lung. It should be emphasized though, that over time there is zonal equilibration with the majority of both ventilation and perfusion (70%–90%) directed to the new lung.

Accelerated Graft Coronary Disease

The large elastic arteries and small muscular arterioles of the lung and epicardial and intramyocardial arteries of the heart develop accelerated arteriosclerosis in combined heart-lung recipients. The incidence of accelerated graft coronary disease in Stanford H-LTx patients is about 90% in autopsies of long-term survivors (more than 6 months). These patients displayed significant narrowing or complete occlusion of one or more epicardial coronary arteries. Acute ischemic events have been the cause of death in two patients and severe triple vessel disease in two others. The etiology of this process remains unknown, but it is thought to be a consequence of chronic heart rejection as in the cardiac transplant recipient (see Chapter 8). The pathologic changes are similar to those described in the heart transplant group and include circumferential myofibroblastic proliferation of the vascular intima. Like the heart recipients, heart-lung patients do not present with angina because of cardiac denervation. Management may include angioplasty in cases with limited disease, and retransplantation in patients with severe triple vessel disease. To date at Stanford, retransplantation for atherosclerotic heart disease (with OB) has been performed in only one patient. A correlation between bronchiolitis obliterans and accelerated coronary disease has been reported and chronic rejection has been implicated as the possible common etiology.

Hyperuricemia and Gout

Hyperuricemia is a recognized complication of cyclosporine therapy and clinical gout has been reported in renal and heart transplant recipients. Hyperuricemia is invariably related to concomitant cyclosporine and diuretic therapy in these patients. Asymptomatic hyperuricemia is very common in our heart-lung transplant patients and three patients have developed acute gouty arthritis. Therapy of hyperuricemia and gout in transplant patients can be a problem. Allopurinol may cause severe neutropenia in patients on concomitant azathioprine therapy, and nonsteroidal anti-inflammatory agents (e.g., indomethacin) may cause worsening of the chronic renal failure. Colchicine is the drug of choice in these patients although gastrointestinal side effects may occur. Minimizing the diuretic therapy may reduce hyperuricemia, and if allopurinol has to be used, reducing the azathioprine to at least 50% of baseline dose is advised.

Lymphoproliferative Disorders

As is well described in other transplant populations (heart, kidney, liver), lymphoproliferative disorder (LPD) may develop in heart-lung and lung transplant recipients. The rate of this complication varies between 9.4% in the Pittsburgh heart-lung group to 2.5% at Stanford. Epstein-Barr viral (EBV) genome has been isolated in the proliferating lymphoid cells by in situ and Southern blot hybridization methods. The reactivation of the EBV is thought to be a result of the immunosuppression therapy, mainly cyclosporine. The clinical presentation usually occurs within the first 6–12 months posttransplant and LPD has been reported as early as 3-months posttransplant. LPD can occur in any organ but commonly affects lung, liver (Figure 8), gastrointestinal tract and at any lymph node site. Morphologically, the distinction between benign and malignant LPD is difficult and both monoclonal and oligoclonal lymphomas have been reported (Figure 9). Treatment for LPD includes reduction of the immunosuppressive therapy and administration of acyclovir, which has been found to have anti-EBV properties. Prognosis varies between complete resolution of both benign and malignant forms in most cases and persistence of tumor in others.

Gastric Dysmotility

Gastric dysmotility (paresis) syndrome occurs in a significant number of heart-lung recipients. It is thought that the perioperative manipulation of the vagus nerve may contribute to delayed gastric emptying with consequent nausea and vomiting. Mild cases may respond to therapy with metoclopramide. In three of our patients, however, pyloromyotomy was needed to alleviate severe chronic gastric outlet obstruction. Upper gastrointestinal endoscopy should be performed to exclude other conditions such as CMV gastritis, peptic ulcer disease, and gastric lymphoma.

Other Complications

Chronic renal failure and hypertension occurs in the majority of heart-lung and lung transplant recipients as a consequence of cyclosporine ther-

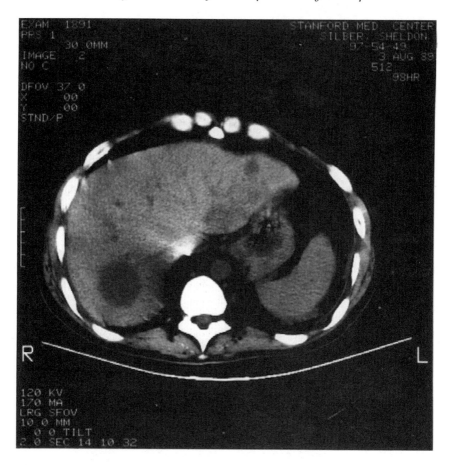

Figure 8. Lymphoproliferative disorder: a liver CT scan of a 30-year-old patient with cystic fibrosis 6 months following heart-lung transplantation showing multiple masses, the largest 4 cm in diameter. Needle biopsy showed lymphoma. EBV genome was identified in the tissue by in situ hybridization. Complete resolution of the masses was seen 3 months later following administration of acyclovir and reduction in immunosuppression.

apy. Hypercholesterolemia is also common but its long-term effect has not yet been determined in this population. Pathogenesis, course and therapy are similar to the heart recipients population (see Chapter 8).

Dermatological complications are also common and include neoplastic (basal and squamous cell carcinoma), infectious (papillomata, herpes), and drug-induced skin disease (acne, stria, subcutaneous masses). Routine

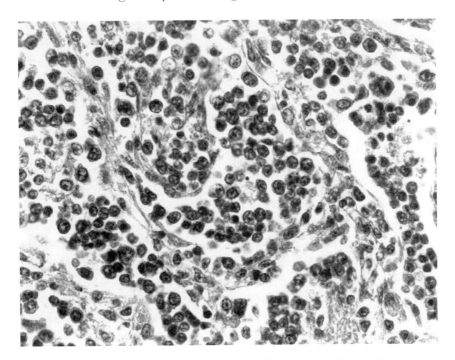

Figure 9. Lymphoproliferative disorder: large cell lymphoma of the polymorphous immunoblastic type that developed 3-months posttransplant in a 37-year-old male recipient. Lymphoma was found in the lung, pericardium, hilar, and mediastinal lymph nodes (hematoxylin and eosin × 500).

dermatological assessment may lead to successful identification and treatment for early lesions.

Headaches are not uncommon among our heart-lung transplant population and pseudotumor cerebri has been identified in two of our patients. Unexplained cerebral hemorrhage was the cause of sudden death in one patient. Psychological disturbances are common posttransplant as with any major surgery or trauma. ICU psychosis, anxiety attacks, and depression episodes, were noted in patients as well as in family members. In most cases, these episodes are transient and related to the stress of transplantation. In some instances, psychiatric intervention is required.

Overall, almost any organ can be involved in the complications of transplantation and the associated side effects of immunosuppressive therapy. Continuous monitoring by the primary physician with regular contact with the transplant team and the consulting specialists, can minimize the incidence of complications and improve the quality and longevity of life in these patients.

Results in Heart-Lung and Lung Transplantation

Heart-Lung Transplantation

Survival Rates Posttransplantation

The Stanford experience of heart-lung transplantation was initially restricted to patients with pulmonary hypertension, either primary or secondary to Eisenmenger physiology. This experience was then expanded to patients with cystic fibrosis, emphysema, and congenital bronchiectasis. Since the first successful heart-lung transplantation in 1981 at Stanford, the number of transplants have increased yearly. While in 1984 the world-wide experience included about 30 patients, in 1986 about 100 patients were transplanted, and in 1988 more than 200 new cases were added. Overall, through 1994 more than 1,700 patients world-wide have had heart-lung transplantation, half of them in the United States.

Through December 1994 a total of 120 patients have received heart-lung transplants at Stanford. Retransplantation has been performed in six patients, with four having a repeat heart-lung transplant and two a single lung transplant. The actuarial survival curve for the 120 patients is shown in Figure 10. Our results have been encouraging over the last 8 years. Survival rates in the years 1981–1986 were 60% at 1 year, 50% at 2 years, 43% at 3 years, and 25% at 5 years. During the years 1986–1994, they have improved significantly, to levels of 70% at 1 year, 66% at 2 years, and 60% at 3 years. Survival since 1986 approaches that of heart transplant recipients

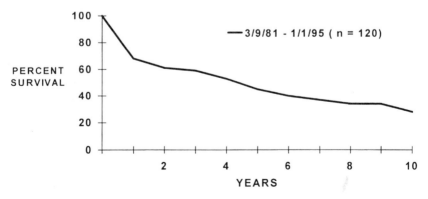

Figure 10. Actuarial survival of heart-lung transplantation at Stanford.

in the same period at Stanford. Similar results have been reported in European centers.

Reasons for improved survival are many and include: improvement in the surgical technique, better selection of donors and recipients, better long distance organ procurement techniques, and an improved immunosuppression. Moreover, we believe that the earlier detection of complications, particularly rejection and infections, by routine surveillance with pulmonary function testing and bronchoscopies with transbronchial biopsies have also contributed to decreased morbidity and mortality.

Causes of Death in Heart-Lung Transplants

Causes of early postoperative mortality at Stanford are listed in Table 3. Infection and hemorrhage are the major causes of early graft loss. In recent years, improvement in surgical technique and the relative exclusion of patients with previous thoracotomies and chronic liver disease have decreased the incidence of severe postoperative hemorrhage. The major causes of late death are infections, OB, and graft atherosclerosis. In the last 6 years OB has been less common and less severe. Infections, however, are still the major cause of death despite aggressive surveillance and prophylactic measures.

Table 3
Causes of Deaths in Heart-Lung Transplants (1981–1994)

	<90 Days	>90 Days
Infection	9	14
Obliterative bronchiolitis	0	10
Graft Atherosclerosis	0	7
Hemorrhage	4	0
Cerebrovascular accident	2	1
Adult respiratory distress syndrome	1	2
Non-specific graft failure	0	1
Rejection	1	0
Non lymphoid cancer	0	1
Other	8	7
Total	25	43

Long-Term Morbidity

Twenty-four patients are currently alive more than 3 years following transplantation (maximum 11.0 years) and 25 are living normal lives. Ten of these have developed OB, with two needing supplemental oxygen and having severe limitation in their daily activities. No patient is currently listed for retransplantation.

Outcome of Heart-Lung Transplant Patients with Cystic Fibrosis

Encouraging results of heart-lung transplantation for cystic fibrosis have been reported in Europe. Large series from England reveal survival rates of over 70% at 1 year and over 50% at 3 years. Cystic fibrosis is not an adverse risk factor for early and late death following heart-lung transplantation. Importantly, an improved quality of life has been noted in these patients at follow-up. Patients with cystic fibrosis may serve as "domino" cardiac donors, with their heart being transplanted into another patient with end-stage cardiac disease, thus optimizing organ usage. At Stanford the survival rates for heart-lung transplants in patients with cystic fibrosis are 65% at 1 year and 57% at 2 years. The abnormal transepithelial bronchial membrane potential found preoperatively in patients with cystic fibrosis has returned to normal (below the suture line) after operation. None of the survivors have developed classic cystic fibrosis lung disease. We have noted that the paranasal sinuses remain an important source of potential infection from pathogenic bacteria (Pseudomonas) and have required considerable surgical attention (Chapter 11).

Outcome of Heart-Lung Transplantation in Pediatric Patients

Experience with heart-lung transplantation in the pediatric population has not been as large as in the adult group, but the worldwide experience shows that the survival rates at 1, 3, and 5 years are similar. Long-term survival at Stanford has been achieved in 2 out of 6 infants (ages 2 months to 3 years) and 6 out of 10 children aged 6–18 years. The literature contains reports of other series of successful heart-lung transplantation in children.

Children generally do as well postoperatively as adults. There are, however, some problems that are unique to children that must be considered.

First, as was noted with heart transplantation, corticosteroid therapy has a marked negative effect on growth. There is some evidence that alternate day dosage may permit some degree of "catch up" growth. Second, there still is no information about long-term effect of transplantation on the growing lung. Third, unlike adults, surveillance for rejection or infection is extremely difficult in children in view of the difficulty in obtaining transbronchial biopsies (small bronchoscopes) and lack of cooperation in performing pulmonary function testing. Overall, the initial experience with this group is encouraging and further world-wide experience is needed.

Single-Lung Transplantation

The first human single-lung transplantation was performed in 1963 by Hardy et al. Since then, for two decades, no long-term successes were reported despite many attempts. In 1983, the Toronto group started performing single-lung transplantations successfully and was soon followed by other centers. The improvement in success rates is attributed to similar factors as in heart-lung transplants (improved immunosuppression, donors and patient selection, etc.) but there are two additional important factors: the introduction of the omental flap technique by Cooper et al., which provides neovascularization of the bronchial anastomosis, and withholding steroid therapy for the perioperative period substantially reduced the airways complications (which had been a major factor in morbidity and mortality in earlier patients). In Toronto from 50 single lung transplants, there were 8 (13%) early deaths and 11 (28%) late deaths, with 62% surviving at least 1 year after operation. Since June 1989, 31 single lung transplants have been performed at Stanford for pulmonary fibrosis (8), primary pulmonary hypertension (4), pulmonary hypertension with Eisenmenger's complex (4), pulmonary lymphangioleiomyomatosis (4), congenital lung disorders (4), bronchopulmonary dysplasia (2), alpha-1 anti-trypsin deficiency (2), emphysema (2), and bronchiolitis obliterans (1). In addition, one patient has undergone a repeat single lung transplant. At present, 15 patients are alive at 9–64 months posttransplant. There has been one case of bronchial stenosis and the incidence of OB at 3-years posttransplant is 17%. Data from the International Society for Heart and Lung Transplantation registry shows that single lung transplantation has been performed in 2,465 patients through the end of 1994, with overall actuarial survival rates of 67% at 1 year, 58% at 2 years, and 50% at 3 years. Single lung transplant has been done in patients with asbestosis, lymphangioleiomyomatosis, eosinophilic granuloma, primary pulmonary hypertension, and bronchiolitis obliterans.

The majority of single lung transplants, though, were done in patients with emphysema (42%), idiopathic pulmonary fibrosis (17%), and alpha-1 anti-trypsin deficiency (16%).

Double-Lung Transplantation and Bilateral Sequential Single Lung Transplantation

Through the end of 1994, 1,344 double lung transplants have been performed worldwide, with survival rates for both adults and children < 18 years reaching 60% at 2 years. The most common indications have been emphysema and cystic fibrosis. initially an en-bloc technique using a tracheal anastomosis was used. Owing to anastomotic problems this has largely been replaced by the bilateral sequential single lung procedure using two bronchial anastomoses (654 performed worldwide). Initially we preferred heart-lung transplantation with the "domino" procedure, but since August 1990 we have performed 17 bilateral sequential lung transplants for alpha-1 anti-trypsin deficiency (6), cystic fibrosis (5), bronchiectasis (3), primary pulmonary hypertension (2), and pulmonary hypertension with Eisenmenger's complex (1). There are 11 survivors at 1–52 months posttransplant.

Heart-Lung or Lung Retransplantation

The International Society for Heart-Lung Transplantation registry through the end of 1994 reports 175 cases of heart-lung or lung retransplantation. Bronchiolitis obliterans is the most common indication for retransplantation. A combined North American-European series of 63 redo lung transplantation procedures showed poorer survival rates than after primary lung transplantation. However, carefully selected patients without disseminated sepsis and multi-organ failure may benefit from repeat lung transplantation. At Stanford since 1981, 6 recipients of heart-lung transplants have been retransplanted—four with repeat heart-lung transplants and two with single lung transplants. One single lung recipient has been retransplanted to date. Long-term survival was achieved in only two of these patients.

Future Directions in Cardiopulmonary Transplantation

Trying to predict the specific changes that will be forthcoming in cardiopulmonary transplantation is very difficult. There are many new developments in a rapidly expanding and evolving field. What is predictable, however, is that during the mid and late 1990s there will be considerable change and progress. The momentum of the 1980s and early 1990s will continue with the development of better immunosuppressive regimens, expanded use of transplantation as an option for patients with end-stage disease, and the further development of artificial organs.

Recipient, Donor, and Immunosuppression Selection

Recipients

Recipient selection for single- and bilateral-sequential lung transplantation should continue to expand. The early results from Stanford and other institutions indicates that other procedures can be applied to selected patients with primary pulmonary hypertension, Eisenmenger's syndrome, and emphysema who would previously have undergone heart-lung transplantation. The increased number of donors available for lung transplantation (as opposed to heart-lung donors), and the improved utilization of scarce donors (potential for a heart transplant with two lung transplants from one donor) will stimulate further growth in this area.

As with heart transplantation during the 1980s, there will be a proliferation of centers performing lung transplants. Since the care of lung transplant patients is more demanding than the care of a heart transplant recipient, hopefully efforts to concentrate the experience to a few large centers will be more successful than the attempts to limit heart transplant centers in the 1980s.

More patients with cystic fibrosis will be undergoing lung transplantation. Previously at Stanford, patients underwent a "domino" heart-lung transplant for cystic fibrosis, septic lung disease, or emphysema. The risk of cardiac rejection and transplant coronary disease can be eliminated, however, if only a lung transplant is performed. The new technique of bilateral sequential single lung transplants poses less risk for airway dehiscence than seen with the classic double-lung transplant. Patients can now safely undergo only lung transplant for cystic fibrosis, and not carry the risks of a transplanted heart.

Our results in pediatric patients undergoing heart and heart-lung transplant are encouraging. Specifically, for patients with complicated congenital heart disease, transplantation will be offered as an alternative to high risk palliative procedures. Long-term toxicity of immunosuppression, which is most apparent in children, may be lessened with the introduction of new immunosuppressives.

Currently, heart recipients are successfully transplanted following hospitalization and support with inotropes, and even mechanical devices. However, in our current situation, lung transplant in patients hospitalized, or on ventilators, or with an elevated bilirubin (as a marker of right heart failure), are frequently fatal. With our current results, these patients are usually "deactivated" so that a scarce graft is not wasted. Many of these patients deteriorate and die while awaiting transplant. By listing patients for transplant earlier in their natural history, and with the availability of more single-lung grafts, this may become less of a problem. However, hopefully more specific and less toxic immunosuppression will allow us to successfully transplant patients who have deteriorated, and avoid the high risk of death from infection previously encountered in these patients.

Donors

Various means of increasing the pool of available donors during the 1980s (using older donors, public education about organ donation, required request laws, organ donor cards, etc.) may have reached a plateau with the leveling off of heart transplant activity since 1990. Further public education in these areas will be helpful in increasing the donor pool, but we will still fall short of our requirement for donors.

Extended preservation of the available cardiac grafts most likely will become a clinical reality during the next several years. The University of Wisconsin solution already has allowed longer preservation, with more elective scheduling of liver transplants in many centers. Similarly effective preservation in heart transplantation could allow for the prospective use of HLA matching to determine distribution of organs to the recipient most likely to benefit.

Not only extended preservation, but also more consistent and predictable preservation, is needed for lung grafts. With current methods, occasional patients will still develop diffuse alveolar damage of the lung transplant, with early graft failure. Current experimental efforts in this area should soon be followed by clinical applications.

Operative Choices

The heart transplant operation will probably change very little. Heart-lung transplants will be performed less often in favor of the single and bilateral lung transplant operations. Heart-lung transplants may eventually be reserved for only the most complicated congenital heart condition, or patients with severe cardiac dysfunction with pulmonary disease. The increased use of lung transplantation facilitates more efficient utilization of donors, and will decrease the spectrum of postoperative morbidity attributed to the transplanted heart.

One option that will be explored for lung transplants is the use of a living related donor. Initial applications may be feasible with a parent or other relative donating a lobe to a child. The adult transplanted lobe would function as a single-lung transplant in the child. Experimental work is being performed on the rate of growth of lung transplants and the occurrence of bronchial stenosis. The living related donor would improve the scarce donor situation for young children.

Immunosuppression

The advances in immunosuppression that will be forthcoming are perhaps the most unpredictable changes. The discovery of cyclosporine A by Borel was primarily fortuitous, and points out the dramatic changes that can occur due to unforeseen discoveries. Although *which* new immunosuppressive will be clinically the most effective and least toxic cannot as yet be predicted, it is almost certain that significant improvements in our current immunosuppressive regimen will be realized in just a few years.

Further work continues on molecules with immunoregulatory properties. FK 506 (Tacrolimus) is a macrolide fungal fermentation product with an immunosuppressive potency 10–100 times greater than cyclosporine A. Approved by the FDA in 1994, encouraging results have been obtained with FK 506 in both adult and pediatric cardiac transplantation and trials are currently underway in lung transplant patients. This agent has been effective as "rescue" therapy for patients suffering from refractory acute rejection despite adequate levels of cyclosporine A.

Rapamycin, another antiproliferative macrolide fermentation product, is currently the subject of Phase I and II trials in cardiac transplant recipients to assess its efficacy in reversing mild allograft rejection. Mycophenolate Mofetil (RS-61443) selectively and reversibly prevents lymphocyte production. Preliminary data suggests it may lessen the development and/or progression of graft coronary artery disease. A multi-institutional study is evaluating this agent as a possible substitute for azathioprine as a component of conventional triple-drug immunosuppression.

The ultimate goal of transplant immunology remains donor specific tolerance, such that the recipient no longer recognizes the transplant as being "foreign". With the experimental work being done on monoclonal antibodies, the pathway to donor specific tolerance may be opening. For example, the use of a monoclonal antibody to the CD4 (helper) T-cell, which is thought to initiate the rejection response, induced donor specific tolerance in a rat model. Donor specific tolerance was demonstrated in a few renal transplant patients at Stanford following total lymphoid irradiation. It may provide another avenue to donor specific tolerance.

The transplant operations are no longer the limiting step in the transplantation process. These new molecules, or monoclonal antibodies will further revolutionize the transplant successes. Which compound, or combination of immunosuppressants, will lead to the goal of donor specific tolerance is not yet determined.

Late Complications

The major late complications posttransplant (transplant coronary artery disease, OB, late deaths from rejection/infection or lymphoma) are closely related to immunosuppression and the rejection response. The current 5% per year mortality following the first year of heart transplant is not acceptable. It is hoped that with improved immunosuppression, as outlined above, and better recognition and treatment of viral infections, that improved late survival will follow.

Alternatives to Allografts

Cardiomyoplasty

Dynamic cardiomyoplasty refers to the use of skeletal muscle to augment the function of the failing heart. A myostimulator is implanted to transform the muscle into a fatigue resistant unit functioning in synchrony with cardiac systole. Over the last 10 years in excess of 400 such procedures have been performed mainly in Europe and South America and to a lesser extent in the United States. The most common configuration has been to wrap the left latissimus dorsi around the ventricles, but many variations have been described. As a result of the skeletal muscle wrap there is geometric reconfiguration of the left ventricle, which leads to enhanced systolic and diastolic function. Symptomatic improvement (on average by two New York Heart Association [NYHA] functional classes) has been more impressive than objective hemodynamic improvement in reported small, noncontrolled series. These changes are often not immediate and up to 6–12 weeks of skeletal muscle training may be required before any symptomatic improvement occurs. Patients with severe NYHA Class IV cardiac failure have a prohibitive operative mortality from cardiomyoplasty and are better served by cardiac transplantation. Transplantation is also preferred in those patients with biventricular failure, massive cardiomegaly, refractory atrial or ventricular arrhythmias, and in those requiring concomitant cardiac surgical procedures. The ideal candidate for cardiomyoplasty is in NYHA functional Class III with preserved right ventricular function in whom the operative mortality is below 10%. At present cardiomyoplasty remains an experimental procedure with further clinical trials being undertaken to define its real role in the management of patients with cardiac failure.

Xenografts

Xenografts are one possible solution to the current donor organ shortage. Clinical cardiac xenografting has been attempted, mostly in the early days of cardiac transplantation. No prolonged survival was achieved. There are major immunological and ethical obstacles to successful clinical xenografting. Natural antispecies antibody mediated hyperacute rejection prevents solid organ xenografting and methods of antibody depletion or complement inactivation are currently being sought. In experimental animals some of the newer immunosuppressive drugs have been used to prevent hyperacute rejection. Nonhuman primates appear to be logical cardiac donors for transplantation into humans. However, the scarcity of higher primates and the anticipated community concerns associated with their use would most likely pose prohibitive practical and ethical problems. Domestic animals that are being bred for human consumption appear to be a more feasible source of organs. In this regard, the pig is under investigation as a possible cardiac donor. Transgenic technology is currently being applied to breed pigs that possess inhibitors of human complement on their vascular endothelium. Studies of pig-to-primate cardiac xenografting using these organs have recently been commenced. The real application of cardiac xenografting may be as a bridge to human allografting, especially in neonates and children too small for support with a mechanical device.

Artificial Organs

Devices such as the Novacor totally implantable electrical left ventricular assist system will be available for adult patients as an alternative to heart transplant in the next few years. Further refinement of this equipment will make this an even more acceptable alternative to transplant. Even if immunosuppression becomes less toxic, more effective, and less expensive, the number of potential recipients will far outweigh the number of donors, and artificial organs will provide a practical solution.

The implantable artificial lung (IVOX, Cardiopulmonics Inc., Salt Lake City, UT, USA) is not as clinically developed as artificial heart technology but is entering Phase II clinical trials. One would anticipate one early clinical application will be as a "bridge" to lung transplant, in a manner similar to our use of artificial heart technology as a bridge to heart transplant.

The solution of using artificial organs for replacement instead of heart and/or lung transplant is so obvious that it seems almost inevitable. With advances in biomaterial engineering, and further financial support of current research efforts, it is to be expected that the current artificial organs will be museum pieces in 100 years, and that the devices will have become clinical reality.

Selected References

1. Armitage JM, Fricker FJ, Kurland G, et al. Pediatric lung transplantation. The years of 1985 to 1992 and the clinical trial of FK 506. J Thorac Cardiovasc Surg 1993;105:337–346.
2. Bates D. The other lung. N Engl J Med 1974;282:277–278.
3. Burke CM, Theodore J, Dawkins KD, et al. Post-transplant obliterative bronchiolitis and other late sequelae in human heart lung transplantation. Chest 1984;86:824–829.
4. Burke CM, Glanville AR, Theodore J, et al. Lung immunogenicity, rejection, and obliterative bronchiolitis. Chest 1987;92:547–549.
5. Cleary ML, Sklar J. Lymphoproliferative disorders in cardiac transplant recipients are monoclonal lymphomas. Lancet 1984;1:489–493.
6. Cooper JD. The "other lung"—revisited. Chest 1989;96:707–708.
7. Cooper JD, Pearson FG, Patterson GA, et al. Use of silicone stents in the management of airway problems. J Thorac Surg 1989;47:371–378.
8. de Hoyos AL, Patterson GA, Maurer JR, et al. Pulmonary transplantation. Early and late results. J Thorac Cardiovasc Surg 1992;103:295–306.
9. de Leval MR, Smyth R, Whitehead B, et al. Heart and lung transplantation for terminal cystic fibrosis. A 4–1/2 year experience. J Thorac Cardiovasc Surg 1991;101:633–642.
10. Egan TM, Detterbeck FC, Mill MR, et al. Improved results of lung transplantation for patients with cystic fibrosis. J Thorac Cardiovasc Surg 1995;109:224–235.
11. Egan TM, Detterbeck FC. Technique and results of double lung transplantation. Chest Surg Clin North Am 1993;3:89–111.
12. El Oakley RM, Jarvis JC. Cardiomyoplasty. A critical review of experimental and clinical results. Circulation 1994;90:2085–2090.
13. Estenne M, Ketelbant P, Pimo G, et al. Human heart-lung transplantation: Phys-

iologic aspects of the denervated lung and post transplant obliterative bronchiolitis. Am Rev Resp Dis 1987;135:976–978.
14. Fiel S. Heart-lung transplantation in cystic fibrosis—overview 1989. Pediatr Pulmonol 1989;4(Suppl):50–52.
15. Flavin T, Shizuru J, Seydel K, et al. Selective T-cell depletion with OX-38 Anti-CD4 monoclonal antibody prevents cardiac allograft rejection in rats. J Heart Transplant 1990;9:482–488.
16. Glanville AR, Baldwin JC, Burke CM, et al. Obliterative bronchiolitis after heart-lung transplantation: Apparent arrest by augmented immunosuppression. Ann Intern Med 1987;107:300–304.
17. Griffith BP, Hardesty RL, Trento A, et al. Heart-lung transplantation: Lessons learned and future hopes. Ann Thorac Surg 1987;43:6–16.
18. Griffith BP, Magee MJ. Single lung transplantation. Chest Surg Clin North Am 1993;3:75–88.
19. Griffith BP. Pulmonary transplantation status in 1989. In Thompson ME, ed. Cardiac Transplantation. Philadelphia, FA Davis Co.
20. Grossman RF, Frost A, Zamel N, et al. Results of single-lung transplantation for bilateral pulmonary fibrosis. N Engl J Med 1990;322:727–733.
21. Hanto DW, Gajl-Peczalska KJ, Frizzera G, et al. EBV induced polyclonal and monoclonal B-cell lymphoproliferative disease occurring after renal transplantation. Ann Surg 1983;83:356–369.
22. Kahl LE, Thompson ME, Griffith BP. Gout in the heart transplant recipient: Physiologic puzzle and therapeutic challenge. Am J Med 1989;87:289–293.
23. Kaye MP. The registry of the international society for heart and lung transplantation: Tenth official report—1993. J Heart Lung Transplant 1993;12:541–548.
24. McCarthy PM, Starnes VA, Theodore J, et al. Improved survival after heart-lung transplantation. J Thorac Cardiovasc Surg 1990;99:54–60.
25. McCarthy PM, Kirby TJ, Mehta AC, et al. State-of-the-art heart-lung and lung transplantation. Cleve Clin J Med 1992;59:307–316.
26. Meiser BM, Wang J, Morris RE. Rapamycin: A new and highly active immunosuppressive macrolide with an efficacy superior to cyclosporine. Prog Immunol 1989;7:1195–1198.
27. Metras D, Shennib H, Kreitmann B, et al. Double-lung transplantation in children: A report of 20 cases. Ann Thorac Surg 1993;55:352–357.
28. Moreira LFP, Stolf NAG, Bocchi EA, et al. Clinical and left ventricular function outcomes up to five years after dynamic cardiomyoplasty. J Thorac Cardiovasc Surg 1995;109:353–363.
29. Morris RE. New small molecule immunosuppressants for transplantation: Review of essential concepts. J Heart Lung Transplant 1993;12:S275-S286.
30. Morris RE, Hoyt EG, Eugui EM, et al. Prolongation of rat heart allograft survival by RS 61443. Surg Forum 1989;40:337–338.
31. Morris RE, Wu J, Shorthouse R. A study of the contrasting effects of cyclosporine, FK506 and rapamycin on the suppression of allograft rejection. Transpl Proc 1990;22:1638–1641.
32. Morris RE, Hoyt EG, Murphy MP, et al. Immunopharmacology of FK-506. Transpl Proc 1989;21:1042–1044.
33. Novick RJ, Ahmad D, Menkis AH, et al. The importance of acquired diffuse bronchomalacia in heart-lung transplant recipients with obliterative bronchiolitis. J Thorac Cardiovasc Surg 1991;101:643–648.

34. Novick RJ, Kaye MP, Patterson GA, et al. Redo lung transplantation: A North American-European experience. J Heart Lung Transplant 1993;12:5–16.
35. Oconnel BM, Abel EA, Nickoloff BJ, et al. Dermatological complications following heart transplantation. J Heart Transplant 1986;5:430–436.
36. Sarris GE, Smith JA, Shumway NE, et al. Long-term results of combined heart-lung transplantation: The Stanford experience. J Heart Lung Transplant 1994; 13:940–949.
37. Shennib H, Noirclerc M, Ernst P, et al. Double-lung transplantation for cystic fibrosis. Ann Thorac Surg 1992;54:27–32.
38. Smith JA, Rosengard BR, Wallwork J. Cardiopulmonary xenotransplantation: The past, the present and future prospects. Asia Pacific J Thorac Cardiovasc Surg 1995;4:8–16.
39. Smythe R, Higenbottam TW, Scot J, et al. Heart-lung transplantation for the management of terminal cardiopulmonary disease in children. Am Rev Resp Dis 1989;20:242A.
40. Starzl TE, Nalesnik MA, Porter KA, et al. Reversibility of lymphomas and lymphoproliferative lesions developing under cyclosporine-steroid therapy. Lancet 1984;1:584–587.
41. Stevens PM, Johnson PC, Bell RL, et al. Regional ventilation and perfusion after lung transplantation in patients with emphysema. N Engl J Med 1974;282:245–249.
42. Strober S, Dhillon M, Schubert, et al. Acquired immune tolerance to cadaveric renal allografts: A study of three patients treated with total lymphoid irradiation. N Engl J Med 1989;321:28–33.
43. Taylor DO, Ensley RD, Olsen SL, et al. Mycophenolate mofetil (RS-61443): Preclinical, clinical and three-year experience in heart transplantation. J Heart Lung Transplant 1994;13:571–582.
44. Taylor PM, Rose ML, Yacoub MH. Expression of MHC antigens in normal human lungs and transplanted lungs with obliterative bronchiolitis. Transplantation 1989;48:506–510.
45. Theodore J, Lewiston N. Lung transplantation comes of age. N Engl J Med 1990;322:772–774.
46. Veith FJ, Koerner SK, Siegelman SS, et al. Single lung transplantation in experimental and human emphysema. Ann Surg 1973;178:463–476.
47. Wood KJ, Morris PJ. Avenues for acquired immune tolerance. Semin Thorac Cardiovasc Surg 1990;2:189–197.
48. Yacoub MH, Banner NR, Khaghani A, et al. Heart-lung transplantation for cystic fibrosis and subsequent domino heart transplantation. J Heart Transplant 1990;9:459–467.
49. Yousem SA, Burke CM, Billingham ME. Pathologic pulmonary alteration in long-term human heart lung transplantation. Hum Pathol 1985;16:911–913.
50. Yousem SA, Berry GJ, Brunk EM, et al. A working formulation for the standardization of nomenclature in the diagnosis of heart and lung rejection: Lung rejection study group. J Heart Transplant 1990;9:593–601.

Index

293

prophylaxis, 156
results, 153, 155
treatment, 155–156
Posttransplant procedures
cardiac transplantation, 63–78
intensive care unit, admission to,
63–65
isolation, 63–64
postoperative medications, 64–65
routine orders, 64
heart-lung, lung transplantation,
226–230
immunosuppression, 226–227
respiratory care, 227–228
routine care, 226
Prazosin, postoperative hypertension and,
161
Preadmission, 31–32, 32t
Precardiopulmonary bypass, pediatric
heart transplantation, 54–55
Prednisolone, cyclosporine and, 105
Preoperative evaluation, heart-lung, lung
transplantation, 197–198
Pressor agents, myocardial damage due to,
immunosuppression and, 114
Primidone, cyclosporine and, 105
Pristinamycin, cyclosporine and, 105
Probucol, hyperlipidemia, postoperative,
163
Protocol, immunosuppression, 100t
Protozoan infection, 145–149
actinomycetes, 148–149
clinical considerations, 148
diagnosis, 148–149
treatment, 149
lung transplantation, 259–260
pneumocystis, 145–147
diagnosis, 146
prophylaxis, 146
symptoms, 145–146
treatment, 146–147
toxoplasmosis, 147–148
clinical considerations, 147
diagnosis, 147
prevalence, 147–148
treatment, 148
Pulmonary artery
anastomosis, 44
dissected, heart-lung, lung transplantation, 210
Pulmonary function tests, lung transplantation, 237–240, 240

Pulmonary infections, lung transplantation, 248, 249–261
general aspects, 249–250
Pulmonary vascular resistance, pediatric
heart transplantation, metabolic manipulations, 52t
Pulmonary veins, retracted, heart-lung,
lung transplantation, 205
PVR. *See* Pulmonary vascular resistance

"Quilty" Effect. *See* Endocardial infiltrates

Ranitidine, cyclosporine and, 105
Recipient organs, excised, heart-lung,
lung transplantation, 212
Recovery, routine, 76–77, 77t
Rehabilitation, posttransplant, 166
Rejection
cardiac transplantation, 102–103,
110–123, 136. *See also* Rejection
active, grading systems, 120t
acute, 115t, 115–118
diagnosing, by endomyocardial
biopsy, 118–119
endocardial infiltrates ("Quilty"
effect), 119
inadequate tissue, 118–119
previous biopsy sites, 119
mild, 115–116, 116
monitoring, 110–120
morphologic grading of, 115t
resolving, 118
clinical manifestations of, 110
first rejection episode, 121
grading of, 120, 120–121
hyperacute, 69, 113–114
posttransplant, 69
immunology of, 99–103
moderate acute, 109, 116–117
ongoing rejection, 121–123
severe acute, 117, 117–118
treatment of, 121–123
first rejection episode, 121
ongoing rejection, 121–123
repeated rejection, 121–123
lung transplant, lung transplantation
mild acute, 244
moderate acute, 245
severe acute, 246
therapy for, 248t, 248–249
treatment options, 248t